UNLEASH THE ENTROPY WITHIN YOU

- Find meaning and purpose in life.

- Stop listening to your programmed brain and discover who you are.

- Become the best version of yourself: Live healthier, stronger, and grounded to reality.

ANA FESSIA

To the Reader:

Thank you for joining my journey!

This book is my gift to you. But it is also a huge "thank you" to life for giving me so many possibilities to grow and learn.

This book's foundation emphasizes those healthy aspects of human functioning. Elements that create a significant and efficient individual in their way of life, due to the recognition that mental health, a peaceful soul, and a healthy body are far more beneficial than the silent programming managing us.

By reading this book, you will find an easy guideline to focus on your thoughts, language, and actions.

I want to start this book, sharing a beautiful piece of text written by Maya Angelou.

She wrote:

"I've learned that no matter what happens, or how bad it seems today, life does go on, and it will be better tomorrow. I've learned that you can tell a lot about a person by the way he/she handles these three things: a rainy day, lost luggage, and a tangled Christmas tree lights. I've learned that regardless of your relationship with your parents, you'll miss them when they're gone from your life. I've learned that making a "living" is not the same as making a "life." I've learned that life sometimes gives you a second chance. I've learned that you shouldn't go through life with a catcher's mitt on

both hands; you need to be able to throw something back. I learned that whenever I decide something with an open heart, I usually make the right decision. I've learned that even when I have pains, I don't have to be one. I've learned that every day, you should reach out and touch someone. People love a warm hug or just a friendly pat on the back. I've learned that people will forget what you said, people will forget what you did, but people will never forget how you made them feel."

- Maya Angelou-

CONTENTS

DEDICATION

To my past, that taught me to be aware of the present and to visualize the future as something reachable, giving me the strength to make it happen.

To my love, best friend, confidant, and life partner, Daniel, who silently and patiently gives me his support in everything I undertake.

To my lovely best friends: Marley and Rocco.

To life, for teaching me the hard way how to become myself again.

To my grandparents, la Nona y el Nono for letting me be a wild child who lived in the freedom of experiencing the world and its mysteries.

To the Universe, for being generous, abundant, and wealthy in health, love, friendship, and motherhood.

PROLOGUE

Each one of us is different. Each one of us has personal theories on the meaning of life.

Some of us have a better self-awareness or a better understanding of life.

Our unique personality, emotions, and beliefs give us a sense of who we are and how we relate to other people.

This book aims to bring you clarity, understanding, and meaning in life. It intends to awake you from the numbness and distinguish reality from the scene programmed in our brains.

Are you searching for answers? Do you have a clear understanding of what you want in life?

This book will help you find the answers but is not for everybody. This book is specifically for those interested in discovering others' perspectives and visualizations to enrich their perception, even if they clearly understand who they are.

I wrote this book to share the last forty-six years of continuous searching for meaning in life. Why? Because you might be having the same questions and concerns I had, or might have experienced frustration, overwhelm, and discouragement.

Sometimes, it is a subconscious self-limiting belief that we are not worthy, feelings deeply seeded in our brains telling us we don't truly deserve happiness and success.

I grew up dreaming of a better world. I was passionate and spontaneous. I often got into trouble because I expressed what I thought directly without a filter. I confronted the outside world many times because I disagreed with what society forced me to be. I lived with generalized anger against almost everything: The system, the way we live, and the rampant human cruelty, selfishness, and apathy. All frustrated me terribly. I felt immense anguish. I thought that I did not belong to this world. After moments, I felt like an alien.

My continuous feeling was, "I need to do something to change the world." I didn't know where to start until I understood that the whole world started with me.

I want to share the knowledge I gained from all the roads I traveled since I was five and help you live a healthy life in all senses.

This book's purpose is:

- To guide you to remember who you are.
- To create awareness, set up achievable goals, and work for your dreams.
- To live grounded in the present, attracting progress, personal growth, health, and wealth.
- To focus you on living responsibly with yourselves, with the world's environmental health, and with all creatures that habitat the planet.

Simply, you will learn pure love for life and those surrounding you.

A SHORT INTRODUCTION TO THE AUTHOR

I was born in Cordoba, Argentina. Since I was a little girl, I was always intrigued and curious about life and avid to explore the world and its mysteries.

I grew up appreciating the simple things in life.

The process of pursuing a change in my life began in 1997, on a cold winter afternoon while sitting at my kitchen table sipping a warm cup of tea.

Like any other person in a particular stage of life, I found myself a stay-at-home mother, raising children, full of responsibilities but empty inside.

This moment was when I began questioning my existence.

I thought to myself: "There must be something more to life than just working, raising children, caring for the husband, and managing the obligations of the house." Those were not small tasks, but they were tasks that made me feel overwhelmed and empty.

I have not come to this world just for that!

I began to think deeply about it. I asked myself questions like, "What's my goal, my mission in life?" "What is my project for when I can focus on myself again?" "What are my dreams?"

I thought in-depth, like any human being does when seeking the meaning of its existence. Thousands of thoughts came into my brain. Of course, my thoughts varied and went from positive to negative, from being a martyr to being self-sufficient. Antagonistic all the time.

Besides this catastrophic and, at times, chaotic state of a twenty-nine-year-old mother, I found myself dealing with internal struggles and a particular burden of unresolved adolescent frustration. I decided to face life without excuses; Without blaming others for my failures, and delving into myself to understand myself better.

The affirmations began to arise to my questions, and something began to make noise inside me. I knew that the time had come to discover who "I" really was and why I was in this world.

I realized my questions were the guidelines that would lead me to understand my essence. Questioning guided me and led me to the moment I was created with a goal and with a purpose. That was my starting point toward this adventure of finding meaning and purpose in life: The place where I existed in a pure state and with a perfect plan for my life.

It is time to discover, question, dig and sharpen our senses to perceive with clarity in our brains what we will internally find by reading this book.

REFLECTIVE THINKING

As evolved beings, we should have represented the subconscious's depth without any stylistic precaution; We should have represented ourselves in pure psychic automatism.

Had we done so, we would have developed the work of the instinct that evolves outside the boundaries of reason.

Humanity should have developed in a surreal way because surrealism is immediate, unreflective, and stripped of all reference to the real.

But, in reality, who knows what is real?

Ana Fessia

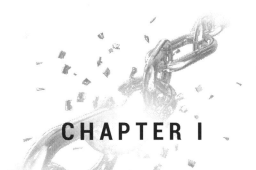

CHAPTER I

Breaking Down The
Meaning of Entropy

Learn to die in life, to learn to live life.

Ana Fessia

During my high school years and the first years of college, I was avid to learn. I learned about chemistry, quantum physics, biology, anatomy, nutrition, genetic, statistic, green environmental resources, and more. At times, I thought I was out of my mind. Later, I understood I was compelling information in my brain to understand the world and people's behavior to interact healthily with them.

I was aware of the programming but refrained from letting the programming manage my life. This synergy generated an internal conflict because, at the same time, I had to interact with the world and be part of it.

I started applying common sense before making decisions. I analyzed everything people told me, and I related all I studied in a practical, easy way to everyday living.

Among other things, I was introduced to the concept of Entropy and the Entropy of the Universe.

What is entropy?

How does it relate to you and the Universe?

By definition, "Entropy" is one of the consequences of the second law of thermodynamics. The most popular concept related to entropy is the idea of the disorder. Entropy is the measure of disorder: "the higher the disorder, the higher the entropy."

Let's start by breaking down the meaning of this book's title.

Entropy is the disorder of the Universe.

Disorder equals chaos.

Chaos equals growing opportunity, evolution, transformation.

If we are one with the Universe, and we live in constant entropy, we have a continuous disorder to clean and organize to dissipate the chaos.

This synchronization with The Universe's entropy allows us to transform, grow, and evolve.

The Universe likes to maximize entropy, which means it will grow and accumulate if we don't do something. As a result of this, we will have massive chaos we will have to dissipate to create more space for more chaos to come. What's optimistic about this? More opportunities for growth, transformation, and evolution.

Entropy is the reason I was immersed in that state of confusion and conflicting chaos. When I started organizing and cleaning spaces within me, the chaos dissipated, and I had a clear understanding of my life.

The Universe will continuously send us Chaos because it's entropic, disorganized, and lazy. But it is efficient. Why is the Universe slothful but efficient? Because it won't waste energy, creating something that requires a lot of work— for instance, it won't create a triangular or square raindrop when it is easier to make it round and save energy. The gravity will shape the raindrop the way we know it, but water drops are round without gravity. This water raindrop is one of many day-to-day examples.

Just as it happens in the Universe, in our internal universe, everything tends to chaos, including our thoughts. We never think or feel that we are one second away from becoming a millionaire, but on the contrary, we believe that we can lose our job or our relationship, or our children can get sick, or we can fall into bankruptcy. We always direct our thoughts to conflicting situations instead of setting our minds straightforwardly analyzing the situation. We have to learn how to let things flow with the universe's forces, which, in the end, will determine the solution to the problem.

We experienced the world through a frame of reference that enables us to understand our world and perceptions. Our brains are hardwired or programmed to create frames of reference to organize our experiences. When the frame of reference does not match our sense of reality, we have a useful tool to apply: The paradigm shift. The paradigm shift is a change from one way of thinking to another, and it can be used to everything in life: your job, your relationships, your home, your surroundings, and most importantly, your health. If we do not reset this programming and give an order to our universe, if we don't obtain energy to make it work using this energy as efficiently as possible, the universe will take care of it for us in an entropic way.

Even in the worst scenarios, there are options to change the way we think.

Let's expressed it graphically or metaphorically: If we are in the middle of the ocean with big waves, and there is no other place where to go, we have three options to choose from:

We can swim and fight against the waves; we can give up and drown, or learn to surf and ride the waves.

We will always deal with unpleasant or stressful situations, and we will have to learn through the process.

Each stage in the cycle of a person's life implies a process of maturation and adaptation to a constant change. These changes are necessary for personal growth.

As you see, there is a direct relationship between the definition of entropy of the Universe and your Universe, which is "YOU."

How are they related?

Our body is our universe, the temple where our soul dwells. We have no other "backup" body or planet where to live. We must be aware and understand that it is imperative to act and unleash the entropy we have created in both. We have to rebuild; recover all the things that we have destroyed. We cannot live healthily in a sick environment.

Both the Universe and our bodies, each from its entropy, seek constant balance. The messages are send loud and clear, but we do not listen.

We must change the way we live, the way we eat and exercise, how we relate with others, and how we interact with the environment.

Some people realize the situation we all are immersed in but just for a moment. After the scary moment passed, most people immediately forget the problem and come back to the irrational and destructive human behavior.

While writing this book, I experienced a process that changed my internal beliefs; I reframed myself changing my life's perspective to create a paradigm shift.

I implemented those changes to improve my life in many ways. Those changes made the vision even more explicit: We can always improve. We can always change. The process of learning in life is infinite and will continue without end.

There is always a starting point for every action and reaction in life. That starting point is crucial when you make decisions that will lead to action.

At one point in life, everybody is searching for meaning. The reason why you get up every day, feed yourself, go to work, relate to others, and exist as a human being has a reason for being, and you need to know what it is exactly.

If you don't know your purpose, you will leave this world without leaving a legacy for those who supported you and loved you along the way. And that includes your habitat: The Planet!

I would like to start by analyzing our lives.

Part of living in Entropy, for different reasons, makes us somehow experience loss. And I don't mean material loss, but emotional, sentimental, or affective deficiencies.

That clutter, that entropic living or chaotic state, made us lose willpower: The power to reach our goals or make dreams come true.

The question is: why? Was the reason the excuse itself, or were we our best excuse for not living or experiencing what we wanted?

What stopped you then, and what paralyze you now?

Please be honest with yourself. Do not answer with a comfortable mindset or excuse. Part of releasing the entropy within you is honestly facing your past, including those painful experiences you might have lived at some point in life.

I wrote below some examples of common excuses we tell ourselves, just to refresh your memory:

- I haven't the money to do what I want.
- My dad passed away, and my life changed dramatically.
- I had a hard childhood.
- I feel too depressed.
- My weight didn't allow me, and my health condition was delicate.
- It was hard even to try.
- I haven't had the time.
- I have to work hard to support my family.

What would happen if you had tried, anyway?

Help yourself through simple exercises to be able to see—and I am not merely referring to "looking," but "*seeing*"—what you have lost along the way. Work to recognize and discover yourself again in this beautiful task of looking within.

Let's start by identifying some lost concepts and rescuing the passion and emotion of living.

How would you define yourself as a child?

Something that might help you remember how you were as a child is focusing your thoughts at three or four years old. Try to remember an episode that made you feel happy back then. It can be a smell, a sound, or someone's smile. You can try visualizing yourself playing, or your mom dressing you or feeding you, having a bath, or playing with your siblings.

Please, write it down in a notebook before you continue reading.

If I had to define a child in its pure state, I would say that they are like little angels with their souls and hearts free of bad feelings. They do not contain hatred or resentment, evil, or envy. Life is a simple game, full of laughs and sweetness.

They express themselves in a simple, upfront way.

They do not deny offering love or tenderness, but they are selective of those who deserve it.

They are nobles, like a king and simple, like a rose petal.

They are passionate and spontaneous.

They are the best a human being can be.

Now, please read what you wrote in your notebook. This exercise of writing and connecting with yourself will help you identify your inner child.

It does not have to be perfect, and it is not going to be perfect. So do not make corrections to what you wrote because it reflects what is sleeping inside your heart.

It does not matter if you consciously agree with it or not. That is who you are—do not masquerade the parts you disagree with. Our mind is mighty and plays a significant role in the reality we live in today since we are creating it second by second with each one of our thoughts. All the time, we are creating events in our lives, even in our sleep. Most of the time, our thoughts are disorganized (entropic) and contradictory. They tend to position us in the role of victimhood or negativity. Our thoughts often spend hours weighing problematic or conflicting situations that we are completely capable of resolving.

The main question comes back again:

Why?

Finding the whys and answering honestly to those whys can create a guideline for a better life experience.

I asked myself those whys in every activity, interaction, experience, or learning process since I was four years old.

I created the following list of some of the "whys" I faced:

- Why don't we try to do things differently than we have always done them?
- Why do I have to follow rules that someone else created?
- Why is this or that person teaching me something that does not apply to his/her own life?
- Why do I have to eat the same food or follow my parents' and grandparents' same diet?

- Why do we have to have a religion?
- Why are there so many religions?
- Why do we have to believe in someone's superior spiritual existence? Isn't he/she/it the energy of the Universe itself?
- Why are children forced to do activities they might dislike? Don't they have a voice?
- Why do we create limiting beliefs that prevent us from achieving goals?
- Why can I not ask questions?
- Why am I in a relationship with this person?
- Why did I decide to be a mother?
- Why have I been programmed to live life the way I do?
- Why don't we make small adjustments to bring significant life changes?
- Why don't I become myself again, as I was originally conceived?

I cannot define which of these questions are most important for you. You need to create your list. Questioning will create a map that will guide you and focus you on what is essential and needs to be changed or adjusted in your life.

Based on your answers to those questions, you have to create your own rules. These rules have to be based on respect, consideration, good behavior, love, friendship, compassion, truth, honesty, care, passion, peace, awareness, wisdom, common sense, patience, and moral values.

Nothing in the Universe was created by casualty or causality. Everything has a meaning, a reason to be, for good or bad, including our existence.

You came into this world to shine, to be brave, to achieve your goals, to make your dreams come true, to expose the beauty of your soul, and to share your gorgeous self with the entire Universe.

You are unique and perfect.

Whoever you address your faith to, God or the Universe, has created you to leave a legacy and draw a path for your descendants and humanity. Each step counts, even as insignificant as it looks. Do not stop in the lack of appreciation of the world surrounding you. Be persistent, constant, patient, and truly honest with yourself.

My advice to you is: Release the inner child within you. We should not stop being children during the growing process.

Analyzing your state in life will help you find clarity. Asking yourself questions will connect the dots and create a map to follow.

Some examples of questions could be:

- What is it that makes me feel the way I feel sometimes?
- How is my relationship with myself?
- What do I consider essential to achieve in my life?
- Why, sometimes, do I feel upset, angry, irritable, reactive, frustrated, deceived, or betrayed?
- Why, sometimes, do I think the entire world is full of hypocrites?

There are answers to almost everything, and it is my goal to help you find those answers.

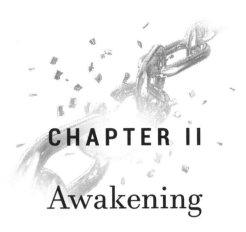

CHAPTER II

Awakening

At the moment that you understand that you are one with the universe, you will integrate the knowledge acquired in life with the way you are setting up your lifestyle.

Ana Fessia

Awakening, enlightenment, change, and rebirth are some of the stages a person experiences after recognizing reality.

At the beginning of this book, I mentioned my process of pursuing a life change while I was immersed in a load of unresolved adolescent frustration. But what were those internal struggles? What was that catastrophic and chaotic stage I was immersed in?

Why, in my late twenties, did I still have a burden of unresolved adolescent frustration? Why did I have all those beliefs of lack, scarcity, and limitation?

I felt I didn't fit in in this world. I started searching and reading everything that crossed my path. Self-help books, self-development books, scientific studies, but nothing brought me a magical solution. I needed a reset process or a reprogramming to find my answers and solutions.

From where did those subconscious beliefs come?

A subconscious belief is a set of programming that develops throughout our unconscious minds. This set of beliefs affects every part of our lives—our daily thinking and actions, how we feed and take care of ourselves, the way we make decisions, how we deal with problems, and how we relate with ourselves and with others—. You will notice that I often refer to scientific terms, and the reason is that if we are based on science, it is hard to be wrong.

Most of the answers we are continually looking for lay in our brainwaves.

Brainwaves are synchronized electric pulses from masses of neurons communicating with each other. At the root of all our thoughts, emotions, and behaviors are communication between neurons within our brains.

There are five types of brainwaves: Alpha, Delta, Beta, Theta, and Gamma. Each brainwave is connected to a different mental state.

Until we are four or five years old, our brains spend most of the time in the Theta state, which is also associated with hypnosis. It doesn't mean that we function hypnotized, but rather that we are extraordinarily perceptive and receptive.

Theta is our gateway to learning, memory, and intuition. In theta, our senses are withdrawn from the external world. At this stage, we observe all the situations and information around us and absorb it like a dry sponge in contact with water.

We deliver this information to our brain from everything we smell, touch, see, feel, and hear from our surroundings, especially from our parents, teachers, bedtime stories, games, movies, and daily activities.

Up until we are five years old, we don't have a filter to screen out information, and it goes straight into our subconscious mind. All the messages we receive about money, relationships, body image, communication methods, the capability to solve problems, our abilities to face difficulties, fears, etc., go straight out to our subconscious.

It's only after six years old that our brain starts filtering information, but our subconscious has already been tuned or programmed by then.

Our childhood programming controls our entire life very quietly.

The information received in childhood may be meaningless in the process of our education, and erroneous guidelines or contradictory references may have made us live in confusion for a long time. Some people live confused for their entire existence, confusing others around them the whole time.

In that process of confusing growth, we lose the original memory we brought intact at birth. This loss is the result of the education we receive, or what I call "programming." Alternatively, "domestication."

By definition, domestication is the process of accustoming an animal, especially for generations of breeding, to live in close association with humans as a pet or work animal. The programming generally creates a dependency on the animal and causes the species to lose its ability to live wild.

Unfortunately for those who believe we are superior to the animal kingdom, human beings are categorized as animals. Furthermore, we are domesticated by patterns transmitted by our closest circle, such as our parents, grandparents, teachers, older siblings, and the society we live in.

The society we are immersed in is constantly receiving programmed messages. Those messages are sent by marketing and advertising companies, the food industry, the pharmaceutical and drug industries, the education system, and government systems worldwide.

Throughout the world, we have been programmed, or domesticated, generations after generations, to live beneficially to the institutions and systems mentioned above (owned and operated by a few wealthy, powerful and influential people).

We start living based on other people's experiences, and we stop listening to our intuition, also known as an inner voice.

Think about a simple task we perform daily: the way you wash the dishes. You do it the way someone taught you without even questioning that there may be a more effective and easy way to do it. Probably, that was not the thought of Josephine Cochrane—the person who invented the dishwasher.

Without questioning anything, we transmit all we have learned to our children who, for generations, will do the same for their children.

We have all suffered the consequences of such domestication.

The programming is what had made us lose our nature, and for which we ended up being someone that we were not exactly. A model specially created to please others, and not necessarily to please ourselves.

I would like to share something with you to help you get into a personal analysis. One of the things I perceived from my grandparents and parents was: "You have to work hard to achieve success." How did this sentence affected me and programming me? In my child mind setup, my brain translated this sentence as: "Success means struggling." Because of that, I lived through life differently than it should be lived.

Let's use me as a case study to analyze the situation.

As a child, my parents sent me to study English, piano, guitar, classical dance, swimming, ceramics, tennis, and probably something else that I do not remember at this time. I think they did this because of their programming—namely, the lack of opportunities they had as children. Perhaps they did not have access to all those activities in their childhood and considered that these learning activities would be treasured for my future.

For sure, they were. But I felt it differently. I felt overwhelmed and fearful of not meeting my parents' expectations. My life was messy, confusing, and it continued being chaotic throughout my teens and for some time into my adulthood. My brainwaves processed those experiences by creating a sense of heaviness and confusion.

I lived without understanding the reason why I had to be the best in everything I undertook. I felt that I had to be the best in sports, the best academically, the best daughter, the best sister, the best wife, the best mother, the best woman. The superhero! A machine!

As I mentioned in the first chapter, after graduating from high school, I studied different careers not related to each other, and I had no idea why I was craving to explore all those different things. Eventually, I came to the conclusion that my brain was to become a knowledgeable library, and my life an endless struggle. That is the way my mind made me feel for years.

The question was still there. Why?

Nothing made sense for me back then. I started at seventeen studying Veterinary Medicine and continued later on with Dentistry.

Years later, in my closer thirties, I graduated with a Diploma in Protocol and Event Planning. Close to my mid-thirties, I was a certified Lifeguard, Swimming Instructor, and Water Therapist specialized in kids with autism and people with Parkinson's.

At the same time, I practiced sports. I did amateur tennis, and I have been a competitive swimmer since I was seven years old. In my twenties, I started training and competing in Triathlon. I practiced Taekwondo and continued training in different disciplines to keep myself healthy.

Later in my forties, I became licensed in finances, insurance, and real estate.

Close to my fifty, my passion for food and cooking led me to become a certified Raw Vegan Chef. Then, I opened a vegan restaurant.

All this fluctuation of varied activities did not prevent me from putting love, passion, and dedication into each of the actions I performed. I was passionate about each one of them and able to create a way of life from each of the certifications I had—except for Veterinary Medicine and Dentistry, but we'll get to that.

Childhood programming created a sense of an emptiness that I couldn't fill.

Over time, I discovered I was highly perceptive of moods, thoughts, and feelings. I was in tune with others' emotions and able to sense emotional energy. That was why I connected well with autistic children, and I was able to communicate with them, even without words.

There was only one standard connection between all those careers and certifications: they were related to "helping." Helping people, helping animals, and helping the planet.

Just like opening a massive door, one day, unexpectedly, all my doubts dissipated. Everything from chemistry, biology, anatomy, physiology, quantum physics, nutrition, pharmacology, cooking, swimming, and all the other things I learned during my entire life, compressed into one single revelation. I realized that everything in life has a purpose and a reason to be.

All those experiences drove me to disintegrate the clutter, the chaos.

I turned my unorganized mind map into an easy-to-follow outline.

I created a clear and straightforward map to have a better understanding of life and its schemes.

If you want to start unleashing the entropy within you, you will first need to integrate all the topics that affect your life. You will need to question your existence, cave deeply inward, and, finally, wake up from childhood programming to better understand yourself and know yourself better.

It's time to wake up!

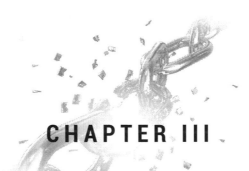

CHAPTER III

Understanding Science, Ourselves, and The Relationship to Entropy

How important is nutrition in our lives?

Do we eat right? Are we knowledgeable about the source of the food we consume?

This information is not trying to induce anyone to follow any dietary style nor influence anyone's diet choices. The ultimate power is always in your hands, and you can decide what is better for your health and lifestyle based on your judgment. We will just arouse the consciousness to see reality without the mask.

To better understand the concept of food, we are going to apply some scientific facts. Those concepts relate directly to how we live, feed ourselves, exercise, work, face problems, react under stressful situations, and interact with others.

Our living is influenced by chemicals produced and released by our body. Keep our internal chemistry in balance is essential to maintain a sustainable, balanced life.

I do not intend to transform this book into a medical symposium or a lecture on quantum physics—I just want to be able to summarize everything I've learned for many years without you needing to go through the same stages. Let's say it is a way to provide you with knowledge in a simple, condensed, and pre-digested way to make you understand more quickly and without so much analysis what you may be experiencing in your daily life.

The first thing I would like to do is to apply a bit of physics and chemistry. It is time to use logic and knowledge to balance our lives.

How do Physics and Chemistry relate to our body's biological functions, feelings, and mood? The food we like to eat, the beverages we drink, and the number of medications we take all affect our body, our state of feelings, and how we interact with others.

Applying logic to chemistry and physics and applying those concepts to our life will help us understand all those feelings of upset, anger, irascibility, reactivity, frustration, deception, and betrayal.

I would like to start with physics and two unique laws.

Newton's Third law of motion, and Charles-Agustin de Coulomb's: Electrostatic Force. These are two related laws.

Coulomb's force is the repulsion of particles or objects because of their electric charge.

Newton's third law of motion is The Law of Action and Reaction, which explains that for every action, there is an equal and opposite reaction.

This law never ceases to act as nature's equalizer, setting in motion compensating electrical forces to remedy every imbalance.

There is a third concept that interacts with the other two mentioned above: The Electron Configuration.

In atomic physics and quantum chemistry, the electron configuration is the distribution of electrons in orbitals. Something alike happens with atoms and molecules (or any other physical structure) like atomic or molecular structures.

This concept is also useful for describing the chemical bonds that hold atoms together.

We are electrically charged with electrons, protons, and neutrons, which is the most minimal expression of ourselves.

The combination of electrons, protons, and neutrons composes an atom, and a group of atoms becomes a molecule.

Our whole body maintains unity between its cells because of the electrical charge and makes us a unit or a body. We are thousands of particles, electrically charged positive and negative, directly connected with the Universe through the third law of motion and electrostatic forces.

Unbalanced charges make us feel a lack of energy, tiredness, or uncharged. Our balance is also related to our internal production of chemical substances like neurotransmitters and the release of many hormones and amino acids that control and regulate many functions in our body—endorphins, serotonin, dopamine, and cortisol, among others.

The primary function of endorphins is to inhibit the transmission of pain signals in the nervous system. The secondary role is to produce a feeling of euphoria.

Endorphins are an essential part of our body's survival mechanisms. They are what allow us to perform at very high levels when we are in extreme situations (fight or flight response)

People with endorphin deficiencies (there are six different types of endorphins) will also have GABA (Gamma-aminobutyric acid) deficiency, serotonin deficiency, and dopamine deficiency.

Some people experience chronic pain in the back or neck, chronic headache, or migraines, or they feel very emotionally sensitive with a tendency to tear up easily. Others are depressed, and some crave pleasure foods like chocolate, wine, and sugar.

Some factors that cause a reduction of endorphin levels are chronic stress and adrenal fatigue, inadequate or ineffective sleep, low blood sugar, intestinal microbiota imbalance, and caffeine and alcohol consumption, among others.

The solution to balance your atomic charges and balance neurotransmitters like endorphins, GABA, serotonin, and dopamine is simple.

Most people don't have access to this information—and even if they do, they find it confusing. For the lack of knowledge, we simply continue doing things the way they have always been done.

Why did I want to explain these concepts to you?

Because I would like you to understand what kind of intrinsic and sophisticated machine we are; everything is related, and thousands of chemical reactions happen simultaneously to make our bodies stay alive and work properly.

When we detect signals in our body or changes in our mood, instead of analyzing what it is, most people ask for prescriptions, consume drugs or alcohol, thinking will fix the problem. Instead of solving it, these substances will further complicate the situation, causing them to end up sicker than before.

When we do not feel well, our body raises red flags through the symptoms experienced to let us know something wrong is happening.

When we feel moody, upset, or tired, we are unbalanced, and this relates directly to the source of the fuel we put in our bodies to make the machine work properly. In other words, it all comes back to the way we feed ourselves.

What we eat is our fuel. The quality of the food makes the machine work well, mediocre, or poorly. An excellent solution to this problem is following an anti-inflammatory and alkaline diet. It will balance all the organic functions for cardiovascular, renal, and respiratory systems; it will level blood pressure, blood ph, glucose levels and balance all the metabolic processes.

An anti-inflammatory diet is a plant-based diet. I will explain to you forward why in more detail.

An excellent way to start is by increasing the number of fruits, veggies (especially greens of all kinds), legumes, cereals, and nuts.

Start suspending the consumption of processed foods, carbonated beverages like soft drinks, all animal products and their derivatives (cheeses, yogurt, ice-cream, salami, pastrami, ham, turkey, sausages, hot dogs, and so on.) Processed foods are very high in saturated fats, sugars, preservatives, colorants, and chemicals that are very harmful to human health. Carbonated beverages have a high content of sugar, colorings, sodium, and toxic chemicals. Animal products and their derivatives are equally processed and contain many harmful ingredients such as preservatives, among other chemical substances, dangerous for our health.

Processed meats such as sausages, hot dogs, and cold meats like ham, salami, and pastrami (just to name some), generate high acidity in our bodies, stimulating the immune system to fight against something the body does not recognize as food or fuel.

Why do I emphasize nutrition as a highlight topic?

Because the way we feed ourselves is directly and proportionally related to our general state of health, physically, mentally, and spiritually.

Think about this for a minute with a clear mind. Sometimes, seeing reality as it is can be shocking.

Process the information you are about to receive with an open yet analytical mind. It can be hard to understand if you are positioning yourself in a closed posture, but the reality is reality, and we cannot let our brain play with it.

When we eat a piece of meat of any kind, we eat a part of a dead animal in the decomposition process.

It's a piece of a corpse, delicately exhibited to make it look attractive and desirable.

When we buy meat, we don't know exactly how much time has passed since that animal was slaughtered, do we?

Here comes the beauty of marketing and programming: meat companies have made us believe in what they need us to believe: That eating corpses is OK and delicious, and have trained our brain to act in consequence.

The food industry contributes billions of dollars to the pharmaceutical and medical industry. They make us truly believe we need those "foods" to maintain good health and prolonged existence.

TV commercials use athletes with white glue on their lips, simulating they are drinking a delicious glass of cow milk to make our brain believe we also need to drink cow milk to look healthy as they look.

On the contrary, the reality is that the food industry provides millions of sick people to the pharmaceutical and medical industry to make billions of dollars just prescribing drugs. These drugs are only more chemical substances that are getting into our system, making us sicker than before.

There is no such thing as a "Healing Drug" in the pharmaceutical industry, nor "Healthy Food" in the processed food industry. Not in today's environment.

Rockefeller changed medical School curricula in the 1900s. The new curricula, which still current until today, focus on training students to prescribe drugs to treat symptoms. Students were no longer instructed to cure diseases. With this, Rockefeller's monopoly in pharmaceutical, medicine, and petrochemicals changed the way we live forever.

Another big misconception created by the food industry and the medical industry was to made us believe that we need cow milk to make our bones strong and to keep adequate calcium levels. Also, they made us believe we must eat meat as a source of protein, iron, and Vitamin B12.

I don't want to overwhelm you with numbers and statistics. Still, it is essential to know that the information we receive is a manipulated and distorted reality, causing us to behave in absurd ways.

Studies of different scientific institutions not paid by the milk industry have proved that eight million women and two million men have osteoporosis from milk consumption. Another thirty-four million have low bone mass, placing them at increased risk for osteoporosis.

Women who drank three glasses of milk or more every day had a nearly doubled risk of cardiovascular disease and a forty-four percent increased risk of cancer than women who drank less than one glass per day.

The researchers also found men's overall risk of death increased by about twenty percent when they drank three or more milk glasses daily.

Why do these diseases happen? Because we are not cow calves, so we shouldn't consume cow's milk. Simple!

I would like you to analyze another bizarre human behavior.

The natural behavior of all mammals in the world is that of breastfeeding their newborns. All the babies are fed with their own mother's milk.

Babies, cubs, or newborns stop having milk from their mothers when they start eating food, which happens after achieving a certain level of maturity in the digestive system.

We, human beings, are the only species that barely breastfeed babies. We give them formula made out of cow's milk, we continue drinking processed milk from cows during adulthood, and we mix milk products with meats and other processed foods.

Isn't that absurd?

Our digestive system is not prepared to process cow milk or any other milk derivative from another species, especially not the casein and lactose contained in cow milk, cheese, yogurt, and other dairy products.

We do not have the enzymes to digest these products because we are not cows or goats. Calves have these enzymes, and their body produces them until they start consuming grass and grains. When their digestive system is mature enough to receive food and can start creating the enzymes to process the food, they stop drinking milk.

The digestive system is mature when the mouth has completed growing all its teeth. The mouth is where the digestive system begins and where the first digestive enzymes are released in the saliva.

After the eating process starts, calves do not drink milk anymore, just like every other mammal species on the planet, including dolphins, whales, and any other ocean mammal. We are the only species that feed babies with processed food when they don't even have teeth in their mouths, and we are the only species where adults drink milk from another species their entire life.

It doesn't make any sense. On the contrary, it is a complete lack of common sense!

Let's break the foggy glass and replace it with a clear one.

All the meat and milk factories started industrializing production after the second world war. Europe was devastated and needed food to feed the troops. Part of the surviving population emigrated to the Americas.

In the United States, Argentina, and Brazil, farmers started receiving incentives and benefits from the government to increase meat and milk production, making the industry grow substantially.

After the recovery of Europe, all the excessive production could no longer be sent abroad. In some countries, especially in the United States, the government began a solid campaign to induce the population to consume excessive quantities of dairy products, meats, sugar, and packaged processed foods.

It gave incentives and benefits to the food industry to use more milk products, add sugar to their product's formula, and add cold meats in their processed food preparations.

Another factor that influenced the production of processed foods was overpopulation. Global human population growth amounts to around 83 million annually or 1.1% per year. The global population has grown from 1 billion in 1800 to 7.8 billion in 2020.

Besides this historical fact, there is a hidden reality people kind of know but refuse to recognize. We create entropy in our lives when we continue repeating patterns without analyzing our daily habits.

Most dairy enthusiasts would be horrified to know the conditions cows endure and how closely dairy cows are tied to veal operations and the rest of the meat industry.

The idyllic scene of Holsteins cattle grazing on a grassy hill that adorns milk cartons and cheese wrappers is nothing more than fantasy. While the meat industry has come under intense scrutiny for the massive factory farm system of raising cattle in confinement, animals in the dairy industry are arguably worse off.

Eating meats, milk, cheese, sour cream, yogurt, ice cream, and other dairy yumminess is impossible when we incorporate reality into our daily living habits and when we get a clear conscience—I'm not referring here to the fat or cholesterol contained in those products.

Calves born into the industrial grip of today's dairy industry have a short road ahead, but not merciful.

Dairy cows are subject to brutal conditions before being sent to slaughter for beef.

Male calves are worth next to nothing in the dairy business. Some are simply left to die after birth. Many are slaughtered for low-grade veal a few days after they are born and will end up as cheap hot dogs or dog food.

The same horrifying scene is seen in pig farms, sheep farms, goat farms, chicken farms, turkey farms, fish farms, and the egg industry.

The reality is, all animals raised for production today have the worst, unhealthiest, and most brutal living conditions you can ever imagine. More than twenty-five million pounds of antibiotics are used annually in chickens, cattle, and swine. Who do you think that end processing all those chemicals compounds in the meat of those animals? Is not another answer more than "Meat eaters."

We have become a disheartened and blind society. But, we have the absolute power to stop this forever.

Each time we buy any of these animal products, we are financially supporting these cruel industries that don't care about us or our health. On the contrary, they sell us lies and products that will make us end very sick sooner or later.

This is the reason I quit my career as a veterinarian.

I chose a career for the love of life and animals, and I was instead trained and mentally programmed to use them. I was trained in genetic engineering to use their embryos for food production, manipulating life without respect. I was instructed to inspect slaughter facilities with blinded eyes and no capability in my brain to analyze the reality that those animals were killed in the cruelest and most unhealthy way.

I was taught to prescribe medications, not need it, to treat the symptoms created by the processed foods we feed them, which will create other complications, making them end sicker.

I can tell you about this because I have seen it all.!

You have the absolute, ultimate power to choose what to put in your mouth!

As consumers, we think processed food is cheap, but in reality, there are many external factors we do not see—but which we do pay for when we go to the supermarket. We pay for the increase in the animals' suffering, the increase in environmental degradation, and the increase in our health and food safety risks.

Our planet is exhausted, devastated, and about to die, and we have no backup planet to move to.

We must get down to work and take care of the dramatic situation on our planet, as well as the deplorable conditions in which certain regions find themselves.

We have the absolute power to contribute to the recovery of the planet. Small adjustments will bring massive changes, beneficial to everyone—but especially to our health.

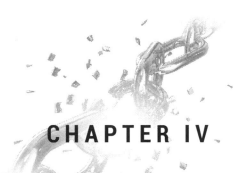

CHAPTER IV

Understanding Nutrition and its Relationship with Entropy

One way to help reduce animal products' consumption is to incorporate fresh vegetables and fruits into our diet. Fewer lands will be deforested to produce grains for livestock feeding. Less water will be used in the meat industry to process meats, and less polluting residues will be pumped into the environment.

It takes 2.5 pounds of grain to produce one pound of beef. Sixty percent of the world's agricultural land is used for beef production. Livestock requires thirty million square kilometers of land to produce twenty-four percent of the world's beef.

The total amount of water needed – to produce one pound of beef is 1,847 gallons of water; one pound of pork takes 576 gallons of water. As a comparison, the water footprint of soybeans is 216 gallons; corn is 108 gallons.

Can you imagine how much we will benefit the planet by changing our habits?

We are talking about just one pound less of beef in your diet; it saves 1,847 gallons of water from waste!

This upcoming week you can contribute to saving the world!

There will always be skeptical people. Some people will refuse to analyze this information, and others will simply refuse to open their eyes to reality.

Some people might say, "It sounds great, but what about protein? Where will I get the protein from?"

The question should be, "Do we need animal protein?"

Let me ask you something before continuing.

When you see dead animals on the side of the road, are you tempted to stop and snack on them?

Do you daydream about killing a cow with your bare hands and eating it raw? If your answer is "NO" to these two questions, then, like it or not, you are an herbivore.

Although many humans choose to eat both plants and meat, earning us the dubious title of "omnivore," we're anatomically herbivorous.

The great news is that if you want to eat like our ancestors, you still can. Their diet was nuts, vegetables, fruit, and legumes. And these are the basis of a healthy lifestyle.

I went through a process to change my programming completely when I realized what I learned by studying odontology. I studied dentistry to complement my veterinarian career.

Cows lose their molars at a young age, causing a loss of weight and lower milk production. This fact is not suitable for the meat and milk industry. One of the solutions applied is to put molar dentures in those young cows.

I studied dentistry to create a practical solution to this problem. But, oh my God! can you imagine how hard it was for me to realize and accept I was part of these cruel industries? To admit I was helping them create more harm, suffering, cruelty, and pain?

After realizing what I was being trained for, I decided I couldn't work as a vet or vet dentist (as I mentioned at the beginning of the book).

The positive thing about studying veterinary medicine and dentistry is that it gave me the knowledge I will tell you next.

Our teeth, jaws, and nails are not designed to be a carnivore.

Humans have short, soft fingernails and small "canine" teeth. In contrast, carnivores all have sharp claws and large canine teeth that are capable of tearing flesh.

Carnivores' jaws move only up and down, requiring them to tear chunks of flesh from their prey and swallow them whole. Humans and other herbivores can move their jaws up and down and side to side, allowing them to grind up fruit, vegetables, and grains with their back teeth.

Like other herbivores' teeth, humans' back molars are flat for grinding grains and fibrous plant foods.

In addition to the human mouth anatomy (which is the beginning of the digestive system), our intestines' length is too long compared to carnivores' intestines. Carnivores have a short and fast gastrointestinal system because they need to eliminate their diet residuals fast to avoid putrefaction inside their bodies. On the contrary, humans' digestive systems are long and slow. It is designed for a completely different diet—because we are herbivores. The digestive system works slowly to disintegrate the soluble fibers contained in the foods that we *should* consume and also to be able to absorb the nutrients contained in our herbivore diet. Besides, carnivore's intestinal flora is completely different than our intestinal flora.

Another detail to consider at the time of comparison is when we ask ourselves the following questions:

Why do carnivores eat first the viscera of their prey?

Why do carnivores hunt mostly herbivores and not other carnivores?

The answers are:

Carnivores need the fermented grass, leaves, grains, and fruits in the herbivores' stomach as a primary source of protein, iron, minerals, and other essential sources of nutrients.

The largest mammals on the planet are herbivores. From where do you think the protein to develop their muscle mass is coming? How does an elephant, a gorilla, a rhino, a giraffe, a bull, or a cow, to produce such a healthy amount of beautiful muscles?

"The most high-quality protein exists in plants." You don't need meats of any kind to have your daily protein intake. Animal meats are the middleman between us and the proper protein sources.

Contrary to popular belief, tons of fruits and vegetables are sources of amino acids essential to building proteins in our body.

Our body requires twenty essential amino acids but produces only nine of the twenty.

The essentials amino acids are Arginine, Histidine, Isoleucine, Lysine, Methionine, Phenylalanine, Threonine, Tryptophan, Valine, Alanine, Aspartic Acid, Cysteine, Glutamic, Glutamine, Glycine, Proline, Serine, and Tyrosine.

It may be hard to believe that the list of fruits, vegetables, and legumes I am about to share with you, are sources of amino acids.

There are hundreds of fruits out there beyond this given list, which will help you build up (synthesize) those proteins with the amino acids contained in them.

Let's start by presenting these beauties:

Peach

Peaches are original from China and contain dietary fiber and roughage, which is the portion of plant-derived food that digestive enzymes cannot completely break down.

It has two main components: soluble fiber—which dissolves in water—and insoluble fiber—which does not dissolve, and it is very beneficial for your gastrointestinal system.

Peaches contain over eighteen essential amino acids.

Durian

Originally from the Malaysian and Indonesian Islands, the durian has been said to taste like heaven but smell like hell. It often resembles a grapefruit and is one of the best sources of amino acids. The durian is rich in carbohydrates, proteins, Vitamins A, B, C, E, and loads of amino acids.

Camu-Camu

Camu-Camu fruit and seeds are rich in nutrients and powerful antioxidants, including vitamin C and flavonoids. Some research indicates that Camu-Camu may effectively fight inflammation, reduce blood sugar, and reduce blood pressure. Valine is the amino acid found in Camu-Camu. It's an essential amino acid, meaning that we must get it in food because our bodies can't produce it. Valine is used by the body to prevent muscle breakdown and is essential for the nervous system and cognitive function.

Açaí

Original from Brazil, the Açaí is also called "The Brazilian miracle berry." Its exceptional properties have proven it to be one of the best sources of amino acids.

Açaí not only helps in protein building but also in generating energy in the body. It is also a potent antioxidant.

Olives

One of the chief sources of essential amino acids, olives, helps produce Oleic Acid, which helps control blood pressure.

Bananas

This fruit should be your best friend. Apart from its remarkable ability to control cramps (thanks to its abundant energy-giving powers and potassium content), bananas are a rich source of Tryptophan, which helps regularize sleep patterns. Very important!

Broccoli

If you like to push this little green tree off your plate, stop and think twice! Research has shown that broccoli is the richest source of amino acids like Arginine, Lysine, Phenylalanine, Histidine, and Isoleucine.

Carrots

Carrots contain abundant amino acids, including Leucine, Valine, Tryptophan, Lysine, Isoleucine, Histidine, and Threonine. They also include vitamins A, B, E, C, and K, among others.

Sweet Corn

It is high in B vitamins and niacin. You don't need more than three tablespoons per serving.

Now, where can I find a good source of protein to replace all meats?

Beans and green peas are two of the highest sources of proteins. One cup of white beans contains sixty-four grams of protein, contrary to the twenty-three contained in eight ounces of red meat.

Other foods high in protein (over twenty-six grams of protein in one cup) include the following: Tempeh, tofu, soy milk, soybeans, lentils, Seitan or wheat gluten, pumpkin seeds, quinoa, black beans, pinto beans, red kidney beans, black-eyed peas, chickpeas, green peas, peanut butter, almonds, almond butter, whole-wheat bread, bulgur, brown rice, spinach, broccoli, mushrooms, artichoke, oatmeal, edamame, asparagus, and the list continues.

So the question is, who has a richer diet when it comes to protein? The answer: people who do not consume meat and who have a balanced, plant-based diet. This answer is correct, but it is contrary to the belief of the majority of the population.

This fact also answers the majority of meat lovers' common question:

What do vegans eat?

Well, the answer is clear—everything I mentioned above, and more! But, let me be even more clear on this point. When I'm talking about a plant-based diet or a vegan diet, I refer directly and exclusively to natural, organically grown ingredients. It does not include any kind of processed food.

Those who do not consume new, fancy, processed, plant-based products and instead only consume all-natural, organically grown ingredients have an abundant variety of healthy food rich in nutrients, proteins, vitamins, and minerals.

Give yourself the great gift of life, all while contributing positively to the environment.

Eat healthy food that neither harms Flora and Fauna's habitat nor tortures or creates animals' suffering. You will help heal the planet, harmonize the ecosystem, and improve personal health and life quality.

Understanding what you can do to help your body improve its health will give you a ton of benefits. It will increase your energy levels and repair cell damage, making a vast and tremendous impact on the quality of your life!

Now, I know what the meat-eaters are thinking: what about vitamin B12? Doesn't it exist only in meats?

Vitamin B12 is generally found in animal products except for honey, but luckily, vitamin B12 is made by bacteria and doesn't need to be obtained from animal products.

The recommended dietary allowance of vitamin B12 for adults is set at 2.4 micrograms/day in the United States.

Dried purple laver, also known as the Wild Arctic Nori (or, commonly, "seaweed"), is an organic plant and is the most suitable vitamin B12 source presently available. It also contains high levels of other nutrients, such as iron and n-3 polyunsaturated fatty acids.

It took me more than thirty years to gather together all this knowledge in an orderly and logical way, applying common sense to the information I received and analyzing the reasons behind each thing.

The way most of the population is living today is self-destructive. If we continue down this path, humanity will be led to live on a depleted planet that will not have the possibility of producing enough food to support us, nor the few remaining animal species that inhabit it.

Everything has been set up in a way that is leading us to massive destruction. Think about the lack of common sense in our daily living and how we treat ourselves and our descendants.

If we compare with other species, we can see the self-destructive behavior we have in our society.

We feed ourselves with inappropriate food. Our diet is from where all the autoimmune diseases, chronic diseases, cardiovascular and respiratory diseases, allergies, digestive problems, and cancer of all types are coming.

Luckily, it's never too late to make adjustments in our lives.

Realizing and understanding how we are manipulated to consume harmful diets makes us aware of the necessary changes.

Plant-based nutrition is the richest in nutrients, the easiest to digest, and is high-quality food. This dietary choice, an anti-inflammatory nutrition plan, will also provide the right nutrients to support healthy neurotransmitter function. Specifically, consuming foods rich in good fats such as coconut, avocados, and olives can also help. Getting a lot of phytonutrients from fruits, vegetables, and herbs is very important to be balanced.

Now that you have the information, it is time to analyze your habits and make the necessary adjustments to improve your lifestyle.

I would like to enumerate some pleasant and enjoyable activities you can practice as a routine to improve your life quality. To keep your atomic charges and neurotransmitter production balanced, an important thing to consider is to keep your vitamin D levels right. Be sure to have regular sun exposure (with the caution it requires). The sun's rays help boost vitamin D levels and stimulate the production of feel-good endorphins.

Look for opportunities to get in the sun more regularly. Go for a walk, sit down outdoors under a tree to read a book, do something you enjoy, like jogging, ride a bike, or simply exercise outdoor. Lay down on the grass, or spend a few hours of the day at the beach. Living near the ocean allows the iodine of the sea to travel in the breeze and to be absorbed through the skin. Iodine is essential to regulate thyroid functions. Avoid the consumption of iodized salt in your diet (another example of damaging processed foods) because it overloads you with iodine and creates thyroid problems. Use Himalayan pink sea salt instead.

Additionally, going barefoot on grass, dirt, or sand will ground your body and stimulate a larger endorphin release, balancing your electrons and protons' charges. Grounding, or earthing, is a therapeutic technique that electrically reconnects you to the Earth.

The second pleasant activity is to listen to your favorite music. Listening to soft music can boost endorphins, which is why we often feel so good when we listen to music we enjoy. If you have endorphin deficiency, I will caution against loud, aggressive, or highly stimulating music until you are more balanced, as it could cause your adrenals to crash.

The third pleasant activity is to eat some pure, raw, dark cacao (only if your liver is in healthy condition). Cacao has a substance called l-phenylalanine, which prevents the breakdown of endorphins. It's a bit like a sustained release of endorphins, except it doesn't last forever. Be sure to get organic raw cacao, with no milk or sugar added and no artificial sweetener in the ingredients.

The fourth activity you can add to your daily routine is deep breathing. Deep breathing is crucial to diminish stress. Taking time to focus on breathing also stimulates endorphin production, oxygenates all organs by delivering oxygen to your cells.

Try taking three minutes to focus on deep breathing. Take a five to ten-second inhalation and a five to ten-second exhalation.

Pay attention to your body signals. Rest for fifteen or twenty minutes when you feel tired. Short naps also reduce stress levels and allow the immune system to repair cell damage.

Besides these proposed activities, consider regular exercise or regular movement a must. It is good for all neurotransmitters but especially for endorphin release.

High-intensity exercise, such as running, swimming, heavyweight training, circuit training, sprinting, or interval training, stimulates abundant amounts of endorphins.

Stretching exercises or yoga are great alternatives, too.

People with an endorphin deficiency will often not be able to adapt and recover fast from high-intensity exercise. Fortunately, they can still move positions and apply deep breathing with regular yoga or pilates practice.

As you can see, all these activities mentioned are simple things to do. But, let me introduce you to something else: "The miraculous effect of laughing."

Find reasons to laugh more often. When was the last time you laughed and played?

Laughter is essential. Laughter boosts the immune system, decreases stress, balances hormones, and increases immune cell growth and antibodies, thus improving your resistance to diseases. Laugh relieves physical tension and stress, leaving your muscles relaxed for a long time afterward.

You won't believe it but, the average child laughs three hundred times per day while adults laugh a little five times.

Be like a child and find ways to add more laughter and play into your life. Both release endorphins and improve your body's ability to make endorphins.

As you can see, there are simple options at your fingertips that can significantly improve your life quality.

Diet influences the release of neurotransmitters. Eat food high in Phenylalanine, an essential amino acid involved in creating DNA. It is also related to brain signaling molecules such as dopamine, norepinephrine (noradrenaline), epinephrine (adrenaline), and skin pigment melanin.

High phenylalanine foods include soybeans, nuts, and seeds—like watermelon seeds, peanuts, sunflower seeds, almonds, pistachio nuts, chia seeds, flaxseeds, sesame seeds, and cashews—as well as legumes and whole grains.

These amino acids block enzymes that break down endorphins, allowing them to stay in the circulation longer. It increases alertness, reduces addictive behaviors, and suppresses crazy appetites.

Now you have a practical, easy, and enjoyable solution when you feel moody.

Summarizing, eat a balanced plant-based diet, and enjoy more time outdoors! Go for a walk to have some sun exposure while listening to relaxing music and eating an apple or dark chocolate piece. Simple, right?

No more excuses. Before long, you will be feeling amazing, experiencing plenty of happiness, and living in balanced harmony with yourself and the planet.

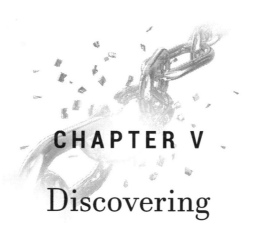

CHAPTER V

Discovering

"I prefer imagination to knowledge. [Knowledge] tells us what we already know and understand. The imagination speaks to us about what we need to know and create."

Albert Einstein

Discovering is an activity to which you have to dedicate time and concentration. It's a process, which implies steps. These steps are the foundation of growing and moving forward.

Start analyzing the past and find the answers to your questions.

Go back through your childhood and remember those fantastic, euphoric feelings.

Rediscover those moments that made you happy as a child. Anecdotes that make you laugh. Memories that bring back the passion and happiness missing within you.

I remember the way we used to play. Imagination was the primary ingredient in all our activities. If I went to have a shower at four years old, I imagined I was in the rainforest under a big storm. During shower time in my thirties, I was probably making a checklist in my head of all the problems I had to solve that day. I spent all my showers as a young adult stressed out and overwhelmed instead of enjoying the warm water running over my body.

When I was five, I liked to make figures with my mashed potatoes. Always something different—a volcano or a pine tree were my favorites! While eating little by little, I reformed the original, imagining other shapes while the first was disappearing.

I'm not telling you to play with your food today—feel free to do it if you want to relive those gorgeous moments. Still, if you think you won't feel comfortable doing it, you can instead serve your plate superbly decorated and enjoy, one by one, each bite, recognizing the flavors in your mouth.

Enjoying life is about making each moment special and unique. You won't have the same plate of food twice, neither the same shower experience.

I still love to do figures with my mashed potatoes!

Discover your feelings, analyzing your feelings. During the day, from the moment you open your eyes in bed till you go back to sleep at night, what are your feelings?

Do you smile when you wake up? Do you feel a peaceful joy inside your body? Do you start the day full of joy, happiness, and gratitude?

Compare the way you felt as a child with the way you feel today. Where did you find happiness as a child? What made you laugh then? What was your favorite secret place? Do you have a favorite secret place today?

Feelings are created in our brains. We can choose how we want to acknowledge and react to those feelings.

There are several human emotions: anger, fear, disgust, excitement, joy, sadness, surprise, contempt, shame, and guilt, to name a few. Each of those emotions can be originated from a different source.

You might like to think you're entirely in control of what you feel. You might think you understand what causes those feelings, too, but your brain can be sneaky sometimes.

It is much involved in interpreting emotional circumstances and crafting your responses to them. Your brain is always affecting how you feel and how you respond to those feelings in ways you are probably not even aware of.

Most Psychologists define emotions as a combination of cognitions, feelings, and actions. What we think of as "emotions" includes how we feel and how we process and respond to those feelings.

I would like to share with you an experience I had a long time ago.

I once attended a coercive coaching group that taught us how to control dominant and manipulative emotions. The group consisted of people of various ages with different problems. Some were couples looking to improve their relationship; others were parents, a few teenage children, married people, single people, etc.

In that group, it was also a girl in her twenties who was sexually abused several times as a child. She wanted to overcome her trauma from that situation to fall in love and have a family. Those particular episodes in her life were causing her to avoid her dream of having a family.

The exercise was the same for everyone, no matter the problem. We had to visualize a particular situation, and then we had to tell the story to a partner assigned for the exercise. The story had to be said three times but from different perspectives.

The first time, the story is told the way we feel it in the present. You express your emotions through crying, expressing your anger, or whatever feeling you experience during your storytelling. The same feelings that had been in our brain since the situation happened.

The second time, we told it as a narrative, as if it happened to someone else.

The third time, we told the same story but laughing.

Most people complained about the third exercise. How am I supposed to say something so painful, funnily? How am I supposed to laugh at what happened to me? Imagine how much some people had to stretch and overcome from inside to say something horrific, but while laughing.

Well, it worked, and everyone in the group left that session without the pain that had deprived them of happiness in their lives.

At the end of the exercise, the entire group was smiling and amazed at how their minds had been keeping them trapped in negative feelings, ruining relationships with others, avoiding sleep, altering their health, and profoundly affecting their lives. This exercise is the perfect example of reframing, cognitive restructuring, or neuroplasticity, which is the brain's capacity to change its internal structure by reorganizing neural pathways, connections, and functions based on new experiences.

Our mind is so powerful that it can create a paradise or a personal hell.

The Chaos or Entropy we know now that exists will last forever. It will cohabit with us forever. We have to organize our inward space to create a peaceful and harmonic place where we can live in a good relationship with ourselves and with others.

Start by analyzing the way you live.

Do you feel satisfied with the way you live today? Are you comfortable immersing yourself in your daily routine? Do you experience plenty of peace of mind? Do you feel pleasure and joy living the way you do?

If the answer to some of these questions is no, or sometimes, you need to delve deep inside and find out why.

If you want to know what type of thoughts you have been having, look no further than your feelings because they give you all the feedback you need about the vibrations you are sending. Any time your mind focuses on memory, thought, or observation, it triggers an emotional response that is either positive or negative.

There are a thousand reasons or excuses we can create to stay in a comfort zone without doing anything. It is an effortless way to excuse ourselves and continue in our uncomfortable, distressing, and upsetting routine.

You always have the opportunity to change things, and it is never too late to put yourself in action.

A way to focus on your life is to depict your life as a picture. Down to the details, make your life bright and unique. Add all you want without limitations. Create a likeness picture of your dream life, and then live it. Do everything you consider necessary to get to the place of your dream. Blaze the trail without boundaries. Envision yourself living, for real, the life of your dreams. Visualize, and then create that reality.

To do this, you first need to feel good about yourself. Learn to connect with your inner self and the world around you. Harness the power and essence of who you are to create and attract the life you want.

Discover the beauty of smiling. Smile more! When you smile, you are sending positive energy to the Universe. There's no denying the feel-good power of this happy facial expression. We are born with the ability to smile, yet we smile (and laugh) less often as we age.

I found several articles that said: children smile an average of four-hundred times per day. A happy adult smiles forty to fifty times per day, and the typical adult smiles only twenty times per day.

Why is smiling important? Smiling offers a mood boost and helps our bodies release cortisol and endorphins that provide numerous health benefits. These benefits include reducing blood pressure, increasing endurance, reducing pain, reducing stress, and strengthening the immune system.

We all have a different perspective on life. Seeing is about perspective. Discover your outlook on yourself, your life, and others.

You will face many challenges and changes throughout your life, but your perspective will ultimately determine whether the experience is positive or negative. Any situation can be either. It is up to how you choose to see things. If you face problematic situations and decide to see them as opportunities for growth, you will learn from the processes and never feel that you are experiencing a big problem. There is always a message implicit in the situation that can be identified and used as a learning process.

In the discovery process, your dreams play an essential role. Discover your dreams.

What do you want to attain, pursue, or possess?

What do you dream of achieving in your life?

How do you visualize or project yourself?

What do you really want your life to be?

Many times we receive messages that we ignore until it is too late. We then regret it when we realized we were aware of it but did not act.

Sometimes those messages come from the subconscious through dreams. Other times it is by instinct.

By definition, sleeping dreams are a series of thoughts, images, and sensations occurring in a person's mind during sleep. On the other hand, conscious dreams are all from your belief systems.

Whatever your conscious mind feeds to your subconscious mind, that thing will happen—whether you like it or not. It is all because of your blind belief and faith in your dreams.

Let's explore more about sleeping dreams. Do you remember theta brainwaves? Well, not only are they the way we connect with our surrounding world when we are four or five years old, but they also occur most often in sleep—likewise dominant in deep meditation.

In theta, we are in a dream. We can experience vivid imagery, intuition, and information beyond our ordinary consciousness. It's where we hold our fears, troubled history, and nightmares.

Sleeping dreams are messages from the subconscious—basically stories and images our mind creates while we sleep. Dreams also can be vivid. Many experts say that dreams exist to help solve problems in our lives, incorporate memories, and process emotions. If you go to bed with a troubling thought, you may wake with a solution or at least feel better about the situation.

Sigmund Freud believed dreams are a window into our subconscious. He thought they reveal a person's unconscious desires, thoughts, and motivations.

Dreams can make you feel happy, sad, or scared. Most vivid dreams occur during deep sleep, REM sleep (rapid eye movement) when the brain is most active.

Sometimes these sleeping dreams do come true. It happens when you begin to believe it firmly. What you think begins to happen in reality because you are programming your subconscious mind so firmly and confidently that it becomes a reality. Your commands, your trust, and your beliefs will make that dream come true.

At this point, my advice is to create a clear vision of your life and believe in that visualization. Take action every day. Do something, no matter how small it may be, and trust, it will bring you closer to your dream. If you believe it will do so, it will take you to the point where you want to be. This is a perfect representation of Newton's third law of motion: "The law of action and reaction."

To summarize, there are many ways to discover and answer many of our internal questions. The call to action is: Discover where you are located in your life to help yourself direct your vision toward the future.

Do this not only to project yourself into the near future but also to place yourself in the present with mental clarity; that it's dissipated entropy!

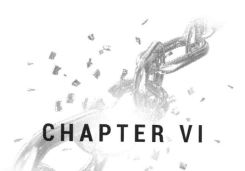

CHAPTER VI

Breaking Stigmas
Building Common sense

---

*There's been a death, no one attended the funeral,
because no one knew who died.*
It was the death of common sense.

Ana Fessia

As you go through this book, it is good to apply what you learn in everyday situations. It can be either a situation that you have lived in the past or you are living now. It will help you to realize clearly and simply how we function as human beings.

We live surrounded by stigmas.

A "stigma" is defined as an attribute, behavior, or reputation, which is socially discrediting in a particular way. Stigmas classify an individual to be mentally undesirable, untrustworthy, or incompetent. This socially constructed notion of social acceptance is based upon identity and association, placing destructive labels on people perceived to be causing pain, segregation, isolation, depression, and irascibility.

As human beings, we have labeled ourselves as parents, teachers, executives, politicians, house-wives, employees, professionals, ordinary people, scholars, and so on. We are labeled based on class, race, gender, and nationality. These labels and classifications create separation and conflicts on different scales in humanity's history.

There is also a long list of bad words used as stigmas to label others— such as nerd, crazy, moron, ugly, dumb, idiot, freak, fat, messed-up, loser, disgusting, nobody, and many more I'm sure you can think of some that are far, far worse than these examples.

Somehow, at some point in our lives, we have all labeled someone with stereotypes. We have all also been the ones who have received this stereotype labeling.

We have created an entire dictionary of words to offend, diss, and disparage people.

So the question bounces back again: Why?

Over the years, I have mastered the ability to sense when people use others to drain or discharge loads they no longer want. I'm sure you can think of a person in your life who takes out their anger on others.

Discharge frustration against all the things that surrounded us will make us learned through painful experiences that this behavior doesn't help us get anywhere.

We turn people into a mirror, which we call barbarities that we dare not say to ourselves.

This discharge of frustration demeans those who have nothing to do with our internal conflict.

We are capable of perceiving people who have these stigmas. We used to feel superiority and power over those whom we despise.

The only thing we achieve with this labeling is to put that particular person in a worse situation than he/she is, only to discharge our internal burden.

We are the most selfish species on the planet. We take from others without worrying about the consequences of our actions.

Think of everyday examples—things that we make every day or see everywhere in day to day living. For instance, take as reference the traffic infractions that are only made because we live in a hurry. We need to pass first, go first, arrive first, but why?

Other examples of the insanity in our society are those frantically actions with an exacerbated degree of intolerance because of impatience.

Every day, more adults—especially parents—are doing irrational things. We have lost the perception of what is essential and the ability to see those important things to our children because we have lost our inner child.

There are many examples to quote. Sometimes we find ourselves insulting someone just because we cannot tolerate ourselves or complaining about everything because we have no control over our emotions.

In today's world, aggressiveness is seen in daily activities as a common ingredient in people's actions. The degree of hostility in a society is directly proportional to the society's habits. Some dietary choices increase stress levels and alter the functions of vital organs.

Another detonating ingredient of irritability is a lack of exercise, also known as a sedentary lifestyle, which generates a decrease in endorphins and leads to the consumption of alcohol, tobacco, drugs, and other addictive substances, creating a negative circle, onerous to recognize, and even harder to stop. Remember: Entropy starts within us.

What can we do to break stigmas and create a better society?

Simple: act with common sense. It is crucial to add a daily exercise to our lives to develop "common sense."

Common sense is the practice of acting judiciously in everyday situations. Common sense is a skill you can get better at with practice by learning to reflect before acting. You can train yourself to use common sense before making any decisions, expressing any words, or taking any action.

Common sense can be developed by exercising prudent judgment based on a simple perception of the situation and self-trust. It is the mental ability to confront challenges and opportunities in life.

Understanding this concept creates awareness in everyday situations.

Common sense is also situational; it is dependent on context. Every situation requires analysis before making a decision. The purpose of common sense is to apply a fraction of a second of thought, which can prevent you from making foolish mistakes. A thinking approach may open your eyes to the possibility that always insisting on being right prevents you from seeing the bigger picture.

It can also serve the purpose of freeing you from rules, theories, ideas, and guidelines that stifle or hide the best decision. In other words, just because someone says so, or only because it has always been done that way, is not a reason to abandon common sense about present needs and changed circumstances.

There are many examples of things we are so used to that we are no longer capable of noticing them. For instance, TV programs; are called "programs" for a reason. They have been and will continue to program people to consume certain products, foods, medicines, or drugs, follow specific role models, adopt political sides, adopt living styles, and the list can continue indefinitely.

The same happens with learning programs in schools, colleges, and universities. The way the information is delivered keeps people from applying common sense. We are trained to become executors of the programming. A few people analyzed the information they receive as education. A few people investigate the origin or the source of information received. Don't take me wrong on this point. I have been the most active person educating herself, but always questioning and investigating the information source.

It is necessary to understand the ease with which the human mind is convinced that an idea is right, contrary to indicators demonstrating otherwise.

Human beings are fallible, and our brains work to provide shortcuts to ensure survival.

In a modern world where caves and sabertooth tigers are things of the past, some of that reactive, split-second judging that used to save us can now land us on an awful locus. Instead of reflecting, we assume;

instead of teasing apart the realities, we follow habits rather than challenging their enduring utility.

These instincts are no longer helping us.

Some of the things our incredible mind is capable of doing are overriding common sense and creating our reality. While each of us creates a reality out of our own experiences and makes sense of our world through this personal lens, for the most part, we understand that our sense of reality is only a small portion of a much larger picture.

Ignoring the facts won't change reality!

For some people, their sense of reality becomes the only sense of reality. They believe that they can manipulate or magically transform situations to turn out the way they want them to be.

Our brain is always overriding common sense, creating responsive, reactive, or associative thinking.

Reactive thinking is based simply on what we've learned through life. It results in us reenacting learned models, applying them to each new situation as they appear, without modifying or analyzing the thought processes applied. This is what I called earlier in this book "domestication," or programming.

This type of thinking overrides common sense and leads to errors in thinking because we refuse to push beyond the traditional associations formed in our minds about how things should be.

We limited ourselves; we only repeat patterns associated with childhood programming.

When we apply what we know to a present situation by referencing a similar past situation by merely using our mind's template without adjusting for context, we're overriding common sense. Even where this template is a bad fit, the insistent, biased mind ignores the template parts that don't fit by trimming them off mentally and only seeing the pieces that "match." Hence, we have our problem solved without thinking it through.

This type of thinking makes us more easily swayed by current popular theories and fads. This thinking manipulates information and makes it confusing—such as the current trend in some societies to control social behavior by increasing fears of germs, the crime index, terrorism, and the lack of job availability.

Without the intention of minimizing the severity of a pandemic created in a laboratory, I would like to mention here the exacerbated global panic created by the media and the confusing and misleading information about COVID-19. There is a lot of misleading information and manipulation to control several countries' societies and economies politically.

The way people think differ abysmally from one each other. Some people appeal to absolute certainty. Absolutist, "black and white" thinking about the world and its people, never allow space for debate. Absolutism is not applying common sense at all.

For such a thinker, the "one true way" is the only way, and therefore for them, it seems like common sense even though it isn't.

Please, try to deal with the feelings that are pushing your buttons while you read. With an open mind, analyze, without prejudice, why you are feeling that way. You will find the roots of many of your problems and the answers to many of your questions.

Many behaviors override common sense, but they are sometimes confusing and challenging to identify.

A typical behavior that overrides common sense is stubbornness. It is a simple unwillingness to be wrong.

Stubbornness is founded on insecurities, fear, incomprehension, anger, and fear of ridicule. Stubbornness is the cause of many irrational and unjustifiable decisions or actions.

So, I invite you to do yourself a huge favor. Disengage from reality.

It's not an invitation to insanity; it is a request to consider that your sense of reality might not be real. What you see is what you have been programmed to see.

Once you start down the slope of self-confirmation that reality is only ever what you see, you will fall into bigotry, selfishness, intolerance, and prejudice. You will continuously want everyone and everything else to conform to your standards of reality and your standards of "what is right." And, you will apply stigmas to everyone with whom you disagree.

By disassociating yourself from this one-sided reality and learning as much as you can about how other people perceive the world and our place in it, you will begin to make room for common sense to grow because your sense will be built on "common" experiences, not just your own.

You can start by looking at your own emotions, beliefs, and practices to ensure they do not override your common sense.

Test different scenarios in your mind to ascertain the practical consequences of applying the decision or action the way you want to.

Account for everything that will happen if things go wrong. And, if things go awry, can you fix them? And if you can't, what will be the consequences?

Interact with others to test whether your reality is clouding your judgment. Consult the situation with others who—you can trust in good faith—will guide you well to gain a broader appreciation of their perspectives and ideas.

Acquaint yourself with your reflective mind. It is the part of your thinking where real common sense resides. The part that takes a bit of a time out from everything rushing you right now suggests that it's time to slow down.

Apply reflective intelligence. It is about stepping back and viewing the bigger picture so you realistically appraise the situation or environment around you, rather than forcing yourself to conform to its suitability or practicing wishful thinking.

After an accurate appraisal of the situation, the reflective mind can set realistic goals, given the parameters you are working within. It will help you to take sensible actions toward meeting those goals.

Rationalizing external signs is fine, but ignoring mismatches to the person you are in the beliefs you hold is a denial of common sense. So, the bucolic scene of Holsteins cattle grazing on a grassy hill won't affect your judgment of what is good or bad for your health—nor will it induce you to consume food or products you don't want to consume.

You need to put your reflective mind to work on each situation you encounter to decide if it will be right for you, your lifestyle, and those around you who would be directly impacted by your decisions.

Another thing I noticed during my re-programming was that we should focus on doing less and thinking more.

I am still working on that and constantly adjusting. It's something we all need to work on. We are obsessed with doing more, all the time, instead of thinking. And while we are running around, frantically busy all the time, we are not productive. We are just contributing to that culture that admires incessantly busy people. Is this common sense?

This dynamic model is about working harder and longer without taking time to reflect. It's an unnecessary rush that makes you run nowhere and ends up overwhelming you in simple situations.

Allocate thinking time every single day, even if it's only twenty minutes. You will notice lower stress levels and markedly improved common sense.

Take a few minutes during the day to connect with yourself. Perceive how you feel about the situation you have in front of you, and respect the space of analysis necessary to resolve that particular situation.

There will be other life situations where you will reacquaint yourself with your rapid cognition or discernment. The previous paragraphs suggested you need to reflect more before you make decisions. Still, the flip-side to reflection is that sometimes, swift things need quick thinking and rapid decisions to produce sound results.

Rapid cognition is reflective thinking under the protocol of Common Sense. It is the type of thinking that tells you that you are not going to immediately connect with a person the moment that you meet them, or that you have to jump because you have a puddle in front of you, or that you need to protect your hands to grab something hot from the stove.

It is crucial to assign time to develop rapid recognition. Spend your reflecting time wisely so you will react wisely when quick thinking is required.

One way to do this is by analyzing past experiences. Common sense builds on your reflection over past experiences. Let me give you an example: If I burned my hand on the oven, the rapid recognition (based on my past experience) will make me apply common sense and cover my hands before touching the stove again. Common sense built on your reflection enables you to refine your understanding of the world and how it works, time and time again. I have met people that never learned from bad experiences in the past and still making the same mistakes over and over.

Some people have gut reactions and have failed to reflect on prior experiences. Reflection will avoid "gut reactions" or fast assessments of situations because your response is based on having taken the time to work through errors and successes of past experiences.

The problem arises when we want something to be other than what it is, falling back into our idea of reality rather than the many facts around us. And *that* is when our common sense fails us.

Realize that this is a process, not a destination. You will have to make the mental effort throughout your life as to which messages you absorb and which people you allow to influence your thinking.

To conclude this chapter, always remember that everything written here is but one source of guidance on common sense. Analyze it, critique its applicability to your circumstances, adopt those that suit you, and disregard those that don't fit with you.

After all, doing so is just plain common sense!

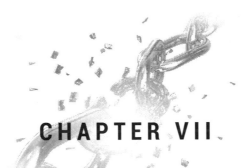

CHAPTER VII

Learning and Putting into Practice: "Applying"

This chapter is a compilation of tips that you can take or leave but analyzing them.

I put it in the book because if I had known all these things in my twenties, my life would be completely different. Not better, not worse, but financially more manageable.

There are many things that we have forgotten to pass along to our descendants as a society. Learning things related to being independent was essential learning when I was a child. That doesn't seem to be the case any longer, but it should be!

There are certain things that every human being should know how to do independently, without having to rely on another person; Things that are related to personal survival, self-knowledge, long-term health, and personal safety. Learning all these things creates harmony in your life and balances the entropic spaces where you would otherwise get exposed and vulnerable.

In quotation marks, "evolution" has helped advance our society in many aspects but has set us back in many others, causing us to lose independence and essential survival ability. The three most critical things I consider imperative to know are: how to fix things, the source of our food, and using natural resources wisely.

We should inform accurately and put that knowledge to practical use when times get tougher or when we need to react quickly in an emergency or survival situation.

Do you know how to cook? If you don't know how to cook, you become a person easily persuaded by others that any food is suitable for you, no matter how unhealthy or unethically sourced. It is no badge of honor not to know how to cook for yourself. Knowing how to prepare the food that will nourish your body is an act of self-love; It will aid in your healthy survival under any conditions. No matter how infrequently you use this skill, it is pleasant and rewarding. It is incredible what you can create on a plate!

I guarantee you will fall in love with the cooking experience, and it will reveal into your life the therapeutic benefits of a lovely and ancient form of edible art.

Do you know how to sow and harvest? Being knowledgeable about how to grow some of your food is an assurance of self-survival. Learn the skill if you haven't already and instill it in your children.

In many overpopulated cities today, several independent projects grow vegetables on the rooftops of buildings. You can have fresh herbs, lettuce, carrots, and tomatoes in any pot-growing right on the balcony if you don't have a garden or a place to grow some vegetables. There is nothing more pleasant than the aroma of fresh herbs in a homemade tomato sauce.

If you are cooking for yourself and perhaps growing some of your food, you will already be more connected with your body's need for healthy nutrition. Eat healthily, in moderation, and meet all appropriate nutritional needs for your age, gender, and personal conditions.

Don't leave your life in other's hands; take control of your own life. You have the ultimate power to choose what is more beneficial for your lifestyle.

Your body is the temple in which you live, the perfect machine that never stops working to keep you alive. Are you aware of it?... Be kind and considerate with it, as with the planet that provides for all of us.

Take the time to get to know your local environment and respond to it appropriately—for instance, by removing harmful chemical ingredients from your home and garden. Anything you spray will get back inside your body and your children's bodies while playing in the grass or the house. Be aware of all the hazardous situations you are creating every time you use chemicals, from laundry detergent to pesticides. All those chemicals you spray inside your home go into the AC system. You will breathe day and night for several weeks all the residual compounds of those chemicals.

Take the time to learn the limitations of your own body. This action includes knowing how many hours of sleep you need and what type of exercise benefits your body and metabolism best. If you don't function well physically, mentally, and emotionally nothing will work harmonically in your life.

Read widely to find the materials that work for you. Exercise your brain and improve your memory. Our brain capability is humongous.

Be aware that your body talks to you all the time, giving you enough signals to take proper actions. You are no superhero. Ignoring bodily injuries is done at your peril. Don't do things like continuing to carry heavy loads with an aching back. Don't refuse to acknowledge constant pains. These are the red flags your body shows you to recognize something is wrong. It seems too obvious what I said, but for sure, you have ignored pain signals more than once in your life.

Analyze situations and think for yourself. Do this instead of digesting the pulp media thrown at you every day, ending up in a state of stress and fear because of it. Every other news item is a crime, a disease, or a disaster.

Start thinking about the reality behind the news feed. Start thinking about life and its happenings with a healthy, open, and questioning mindset.

Induction by manipulation is an old tactic used by the media to direct you to do things without letting you think about your actions' consequences. Media manipulates your consumption and spending habits, including how you dress, what you eat, what you drink, what over-the-counter medications you need, what car you want to drive, and overall how you feel you "have" to live.

We have turned into zombies. We don't think or analyze any of the information sent subliminally to our brain. We act irrationally!.

Maybe you never thought about this, and I'm conscious that we live in modern and evolving times, but consumerism has led us to discard things, even if those things have been used for a short time. In a world very dependent on eliminating articles rather than repairing them, we add more garbage to the Earth, and we are in debt to ourselves.

Because of those who manufacture articles with built-in obsolescence, we spend money buying and replacing things because we have lost the ability to repair things. Of course, there will be things that can't be fixed—but we have gotten used to discarding instead of taking a look to see if they are fixable.

Learning to fix or repair clothes, appliances, household objects, automobile engines, install a plug or a switch, change a tire, and many other essential elements for our daily functioning is liberating and a meaningful way to exercise our common sense.

I'm not telling you to do it every day, neither to be part of your living style. But if you are in a situation one day, and you know about these things, you will be able to apply this knowledge and solve the problem.

As I mentioned already, social media have the goal to hit us with empty and confusing consumer content to induce our unconscious minds. All this massive consumerism leads us to end financially broken. But there is a reason why.

Nowhere are we taught how to manage personal finances, budget, and not spend more than we earn. This information is essential for financial freedom. Spend wisely based on what you have.

Not all of us have access to financial education. Lack of knowledge leaves us in a bad position to make essential financial decisions.

Unfortunately, many people use credit cards thinking that the credit card has money in it to pay for their expenses. They manage to forget about this frequent overspending and later behave as if their bulging credit card debt is a complete surprise.

Overspending is an irrational habit, as is hiding unopened bills in the back of a drawer.

You should be reining in spending with a budget and self-restraint.

Something I learned in finance is that we always have to carry cash instead of cards. It will help you realize how much money you have taken out of your bank account at the end of the day. Save the credit cards only for emergencies, and build a cash emergency fund. There will be situations where you won't be able to use debit or credit cards.

The best way to grow financially is the following formula: Save one-third of each paycheck or your income for projects, dreams, or vacations, and one-third for retirement. Invest this money in a retirement plan, Roth IRA, or mutual fund. The younger you start saving and investing in your future, the safer you will be when it comes to retirement. Diversify your investments wisely, from real estate to bonds, and stocks, to create passive income. Consult an honest and trusted financial advisor and make sure to get all important financial decisions and agreements in writing, from loans to sales—you must be very careful when it comes to money.

Learn how to plan, so you're not doing things haphazardly, more expensively than needed, or without an idea of the consequences.

Forward-thinking is always a sign of good common sense, as it can review the consequences of different outcomes.

Unfortunately, money has become a manipulative instrument from which we cannot liberate for now.

Everything around our life is related to money and directed by money, limiting us sometimes to make decisions that bring good changes into our life. But there is a way out: "Being resourceful."

Knowing how to be resourceful will help you instantly solve many different situations presented in life. Resourcefulness is the art of "making do;" it's about taking small things and making them go a long way with a little imagination and constant work: persistence and perseverance. Two attributes we can develop in time.

It's about being able to thrive under challenging conditions and still prosper without feeling deprived. Resourcefulness is a key, and again, it's a skill that liberates you from consuming yourself to live a good life.

Always remember that human beings are social creatures. Stay connected with your community and be a part of your community. Unfortunately, the way we live today—hidden behind electronic devices and lately with a mask in our face—makes many people prefer to bunker down and remain aloof to those around them.

Interact with others in your community, open yourself up to sharing, and being generous. These are beautiful attributes, and they are qualities not everybody develops or applies.

There may be people reading this book who think what I am expressing is very obvious and logical, and there may be others who believe it is naive. But not everyone has had the resources to find answers to their questions or the opportunity to practice and develop common sense, open up to new possibilities, or expose themselves to live new experiences.

Even in situations where we acknowledge something can happen if we do not take precautions, we sometimes fail. We are simply human beings, and we often downplay everyday situations that require our attention.

Value your life because there are not two opportunities to live. Not, at least, two lives that you can remember if you believe in reincarnation. You will forget all these life experiences in your next life.

Avoid risky situations that put you unnecessarily in danger. Whether you're in public or at home, safety is a matter of common sense. It seems obvious, but a lot of accidents happen because someone has not applied common sense. How many times have you burned yourself in the kitchen on hot surfaces? It's not just because "accidents happen," it's because we do not prevent them. It only takes a fraction of a second of distraction for something to happen. Put thinking thought into action before anything harmful happens. Doing so will avert problems altogether.

Take the necessary time to reply to a text message when you are not driving a car or riding a bicycle. I have seen people texting while cycling, and I have been in groups of cyclists who have been hit by a car whose driver was texting.

Let your friends know that you will not be available to text for a few minutes, or just wait until you are in a safe situation to use your phone, put on makeup, eat, or do anything else beyond merely driving. The car is not the right place for you to do anything else more than drive. Common sense, right?

Put new thinking habits into place. Take popular theories and put them behind how you think. Add this understanding to the active ways in which you can use your common sense.

If you have noticed, all the situations and actions mentioned above arise when we don't apply common sense. Instead, we act irrationally, creating chaos and entropic situations in our lives.

Restore your sense of relying on your innovative thinking processes.

Keep your practical intelligence and common sense in top shape. Stretch yourself until you become an elastic, flexible thinker. Practicing mental flexibility is the ability to stay open-minded and listen to other people's notions and ideas. Even if they dislike you, scare you, or betray and derail your thinking, it does you good to practice mental elasticity and to stretch yourself beyond the things you think you know already.

Don't let pessimism drive you. Use affirmative thinking to positively perceive yourself and others, always seeking to see the best in others and yourself. Make a consistent decision about who or what will influence you. Define who is worthy of your time. Mental work is required to maintain an affirmative, conscious mindset. It is challenging but rewarding.

Be kind and inspiring to others to do the same. Empower them for their right actions. These aren't simplistic affirmations.

Being human is to have or develop the capability to recognize and connect with others deeply as the social creatures we are by nature. Rely on semantic sanity. Use positive talking. It is the way to projecting yourself and others to a more elevated space of relationship. It is about using language to support clear thinking, freed from dogmas, beliefs, or doctrines.

Practicing neutrality and learn how to value others' ideas is a concept that leads you to accept new ideas rather than immediately blocking them in your head as unfamiliar, insane, or undoable.

How do you know they don't match your viewpoint if you haven't worked through them? Valuing ideas epitomizes the need to reflect. Without adequate time for reflection, you will fail to come up with your ideas.

If you put in the harshness of thinking things through carefully for yourself and learning all you can about the world and others' thoughts about the world, you are well placed. You don't have to be highly educated; you just have to be open-minded and curious.

Summarizing this chapter, life itself is a never-ending learning process. You can rely on others' knowledge to do things, trust others in deciding about your life, or get knowledgeable yourself for self-survival.

Now that we are more aware of how our mind biases things, situations, and experiences, we must clean and fix all the issues we have identified to live consciously and connected to reality.

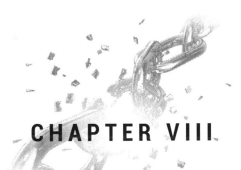

CHAPTER VIII

Identifying, Cleaning, and Fixing Relationships

This book reflects some of my life experiences and journey to pursue a balanced harmony with the universe, knowing that we are immersed in constant entropy. Identify what parts of it make sense to you, analyzing the content, and making your conclusions. You don't have to agree with everything expressed in this book.

This chapter is about identifying, cleaning, and fixing our inner relationship with ourselves and our relationships with others and the world. It could be one of the most challenging tasks to go through, but that depends on how you allow your mind to interact with the situations presented.

Before trying to fix your life's loopholes and how you relate with others, you need to figure out the source of the problems.

Identifying who you are and where you've come from requires you to remain open-minded and alert. You need to listen to your most resonant inner voice.

There will be a load of information that needs to be processed. This action will lead you to develop an awareness of who you are and keep alert to your mind sabotages to execute and keep you confused.

The inner place you are accustomed to residing in today has become too small to move and expand, but it is comfortable enough to don't have the restlessness to move aside, observe in detail, and deep clean it.

It is time to deep dredge our lives for a healthy existence. We are talking about awakening from the numbness of being accustomed or acclimatized to situations or interpersonal relationships that we acknowledge are wrong, harm us, or are toxic. It is not an easy task to perform. In the first place, it requires awareness that this numbness exists, and secondly, it requires recognizing that we must take action. It is the most critical part of our entropy or chaotic existence: "Relationships."

Deciding to take the first step toward cleaning inner spaces requires courage and determination. But furthermore—and beyond all the expressions in this chapter—whatever action you take must be your own decision, and it has to be analyzed in depth before any action is taken.

It is not quite an exercise; it is more of an introspective search. The main reason to do that is to deeply clean your inner space, starting with identifying toxic relationships.

Ask yourself what your relationships with others are like, starting with your closest circle. For example, this may be family members who live with you and interact with you and each other in your everyday routine. This introspective search will help you identify hidden problems in the relationship.

Most members of a family live together without questioning their coexistence.

We were born into that family, and, by nature, we belong to that tribe. We are accustomed to how we dialogue, the way we exchange ideas, and how we share activities. If we disagree with another's thinking, depending on the nature of the relationship, in that case, we can either express our thinking or remain in the healthy silence of acceptance, digesting the idea imposed by the strongest in the tribe and continue our way.

Our closest relationships easily persuade us because we naturally trust each other. We do not have a reference to compare them to because they are the only family we have.

The members of a healthy family interact with each other in respectful, harmonious, and mutual tolerance. Unfortunately, not all families are healthy because we are not all emotionally and mentally balanced.

Toxic relationships between family members can destroy one or both members involved in the toxic relationship. We can spend years sacrificing our mental and emotional health in abusive relationships under the notion that "we have to" because they are family.

Ending a familial relationship and cutting ties with family members is one of the most difficult decisions we can face in life. Family members are just people, and they are not always emotionally or mentally healthy people. If these people were not family, we would never choose them to be part of our lives due to their awful treatment of us.

Always keep in mind and clearly understand that you are one hundred percent responsible for your own decisions. You can not appoint anyone around you to be liable for any of the decisions you take in your life, be it a simple meal choice or a huge and significant change in your life.

Through all the roads traveled in my life, I have gained the wisdom to recognize specific patterns of manipulative and irrational behaviors.

I can't say I'm a master or an experienced professional in this matter, but yes, I am knowledgeable enough to discuss this topic effectively.

In my humble opinion, based on my experience, when a relationship is founded on any kind of abuse—mental, physical, sexual, verbal, or emotional—or when the relationship is based on manipulation—overt or covert—we can be sure we are being used, abused, and involved in a toxic relationship.

If you live in a constant, stressful state of anxiety and fear, never knowing or predicting how the person will react against you, any engagement you have with this person should end.

It is time to love yourself enough to let go. Be brave enough to go far from that person and the relationship.

No matter if the relationship is with any family member—husband, wife, son, daughter, siblings—or if it is with a friend. It is time to terminate a relationship when the only contact you have with them is harmful and destructive.

Toxic interactions or relationships are those in which each interaction only serves to bring you down and emotionally destabilize you, making you feel you are not good enough. It will diminish you or make you think you haven't done enough for them.

When the relationship creates so much stress that it affects other important areas of your life, like your relationships with other people, your work, or your home, it must end.

The perception of your emotions is that you are caught up in defending yourself and wanting to explain yourself all the time.

You will find yourself talking about the chaos of your relationships with other people all the time, obsessed with gossip about you, always trying to correct the wrong information.

When you feel you are continually ostracized to the point you are losing sleep, you are becoming poisoned with their toxicity. Gossiping serves one member to get others to gang up on him/her, leaving you defenseless against false beliefs. As it is said: divide and conquer.

There is usually a leader gathering others and creating confusion. You begin to wonder whether it is *you* that is the problem.

Under these circumstances, the relationship's problem is entirely all about the other person. There is no real reason why the other person cannot make any effort toward the health of the relationship with you.

One-sided relationships are set up for failure. When you realize there is never going to be "enough" place for you to reach in the relationship, you need to let go and start to focus on your healing.

Another example is when the relationship is only about borrowing, needing money, or abusively taking what rightfully belongs to you. It is a common type of relationship manifested by abusive sons or daughters with one of their parents. They tend to team-up with one of the parents and manipulate the other. It is frequently seen in the family relationships of divorced parents.

When speculative games dominate the relationship, such as the silent treatment, indifference, blame-games, no-win arguments spinning around on you, etc., there is no point in continuing in this battle.

Verbal warfare is never the place where you will convince them of anything, and these kinds of verbal interactions are set up to end in their favor. If these are the negative consequences you're receiving each time this person doesn't get their way, it is time to let go. You will always love your family members, but you won't allow them to harm your feelings with their behavior. It is not about to stop loving; it is about to stop allowing.

We can improve relationships primarily through communication. Knowing how to communicate effectively can often be overwhelming, especially between couples. Other types of relationships grant more space for understanding.

One of the most common negative patterns is the cycle of criticism and defensiveness, more often between couples and other close relationships. Usually, it happens when you hear something you perceive as an attack or criticism from the other person involved in the relationship, which leads you immediately to defend yourself.

This pattern sets both of you up not to be heard. As soon as you start to defend your position, you've lost the opportunity to understand the other person. Even if you feel under attack or think you hear criticism, try to understand the other person's thoughts and feelings before you respond. Seek to understand more before trying to be understood.

In many cases, communication starts speeding up in tone, volume, and vocabulary.

Many problems get out of control because once this belligerent storm of criticism and defense is underway, the interaction often moves quickly. When your communication accelerates, you may lose a lot of important information the other party is expressing. This rapid pace also increases the discussion's volatility, making it difficult to keep the conversation hushed. Try to slow down the communication to listen to the other party.

As soon as you notice, the conversation starts speeding, push the brakes intentionally, and slow down the dynamic.

Make sure the other party knows you want to understand what he/she is saying. It helps deactivate reactivity and allows you to continue communicating in an adult-to-adult manner.

A little tip here: "Practice curiosity." Being curious about the other's perspective is easier said than done when you feel blamed, criticized, or attacked. Still, one of the best things you can do in such circumstances is to be curious about the other party's perspective. This action disarms the tension positively and immediately helps decrease the growing argument between both. Being curious leads you to learn new things about the other person and support your conversation move toward a resolution.

You may still disagree with the other's perspective while remaining curious and interested in how your vision is different from others'.

Work to recognize your emotional triggers and learn to calm down. Knowing your emotional triggers allows you to be aware of when the potential for their activation is present. We all bring "baggage" to our relationships, from our childhood, previous relationships, life experiences, and, of course, our family of origin. There is no such thing as a person who is "free of baggage." However, you can use your knowledge of your hot spots to know when they are likely to be activated.

Practicing self-observation can help you discover how some conversations with the other person in the relationship had touched something in the past that is not related to the actual person. This understanding can help both to be less reactive at the moment.

Use empathy to encourage a closer connection. Empathy is the fuel of good relationships. Being empathetic is imagining yourself walking in another's shoes and seeing the world from their perspective. Empathically responding to others facilitates a deeper bond and creates a strong sense of security and trust between both parties. However, when you feel attacked, this is the last thing you want to do. It requires you to get out of yourself and begin to appreciate a reality different from yours.

My grandmother always told me that over the years comes experience, and with experience comes wisdom. There is also a saying that "knowledge is gained through years of experience." Over the past fifty-two years, life's experiences helped me develop an extensive analytical vision on sharing a relationship with another person. It's not always easy, and it's not always feasible.

The ideal would be to have a leisurely and wise vision on how to share a relationship.

Practicing empathy does not mean that you have to give up entirely and forsaking what you want or renouncing your reality. It just means that you must suspend your perspective, even momentarily, so you can appreciate the smallest part of how others see things.

Start small, even if you only imagine between one and five percent of what the other party feels, and then take advantage of that. The other party will feel the change and lower their guard a little, opening the possibility of a better connection.

When you genuinely listen to the other party, you listen to their hidden need or unfulfilled emotions. There is always some need, desire, or emotion not spoken, not satisfied behind this blubbering. The challenge for you is to go below the open complaint and see if you can uncover the hidden emotion. Discovering this emotion can avoid anger, irritation, or resentment from the surface and eliminate the central feeling that needs to be validated.

Being a good listener is not an easy task since it requires you to figuratively get away from the current conflict to observe what is *not* expressed. It also requires you to suspend your reactivity and defensiveness to connect with the other's deepest needs.

Pause for a moment, and see if you can feel what else in the conversation the other person is not expressing. It can be a complaint or feels criticized or blamed. Be aware that the other part can not share the full picture of the problem with you. Listen carefully to this and use your curiosity to discover what else is not being shared openly.

My favorite quote in this matter is: "There are always two parties needed for a fight."

Anticipate issues before they become an argument. Many problems in relationships could have been dealt with much earlier but weren't. Avoiding talking about small statements can often lead to unresolved issues expanding over time, exploding, and becoming more significant than initially. You may not want to create a problem when things seem to be going well. You may believe that nothing good comes from raising complaints or issues, but the reality is that doing so helps both parties grow in their relationship in a healthy manner.

Get into the habit of naming and flagging issues with each other early on, always from a space of mutual respect over time. This structure will help both parties involved in the relationship feel more confident about effectively dealing with conflicts and disagreements.

In any relationship, communication requires constant attention. Do not stress out. I recommend you start with the basics and establish communication and connection rituals to ensure the longevity of your love with your couple, your children, your friends, your siblings, and the connections with each other.

Fixing is the next step. First, discover the reasons for entropic relationships.

If you have noticed changes in your behavior—especially if you are moody or feel you have lost your inner peace—try to find out the possible reasons behind it.

As you are well aware of your likes and dislikes, finding out the cause and fixing the problem won't be a difficult job—so long as you are deeply honest with yourself and put the effort and dedication into assigning time for this purpose.

Improve communication with yourself. Try to be a good self-listener. Make sure that you always lend an ear to what your inner voice has to say. You can't be the only one talking all the time, silencing your inner voice. Let your inner voice express itself freely. You will feel self-valued, and you will give yourself a better chance of understanding issues.

Bury your past and the painful situations that have happened to you. Focus on your present, and fix the issues that are spoiling it. You can never be happy focusing on the past. Forgive the past and the people involved. It helps you save your future relationships, starting with the relationship you have with yourself. Fixing your problems is all about understanding and giving yourself a second chance. Forget what happened in the past and start all over; it will help declutter your mind and prevent the past from clouding your judgments.

Learn to compromise. Commit to yourself. Being in a serious relationship with yourself and others is all about compromises. You can't always have things your way. It will be better to emotionally grow healthier and stronger if sometimes you admit others' ways were right.

It is more about spending quality time with yourself and your inner Entropy. Even doing something you're not fond of can be positive—give new things a try. Dissipate the chaos by trying new things that make you feel good. Get to know other facets of yourself. The secret is that spending more time with yourself will guide you to find out the real problem. Then, you can look for a solution accordingly.

Learn to communicate. Communication is a skill we have to develop and polish to perfection. It will never be perfect, but we have to make our best effort for ourselves and our surroundings.

Don't expect others to guess your thoughts and emotions. Instead, be vocal about your feelings. If you don't talk openly about your expectations, they will never be able to understand. As a result, a communication gap will form too deep to fill, giving space for conflicting emotions to root.

Do not react if the response you receive is not the one expected. Try your best to understand what the other person is trying to communicate.

Be tolerant, patient, respectful, and peaceful. Become a master in the art of communicating with others learning to communicate with yourself first.

In conclusion, fixing the loopholes of your life dissipate chaos, and unleash entropy. Start with the way you relate with yourself and others. These relationships must be healthy and based on respect.

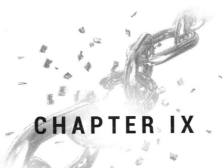

CHAPTER IX

Redefining Who You Are

Understanding Self Identity.

Life, people, events, and circumstances are consistently random and unpredictable. They are certainly not designed with our best interests in mind all the time. Due to the natural entropy we live immersed in, the question, "Who I am?" is the question everyone at some point will ask themselves.

Indeed, many organizations, religions, and self-help Gurus have attempted to provide an answer to that question on your behalf. Still, their answers come from philosophies developed in the bronze age and no longer will be practical assistance when it comes to an understanding—and more importantly, changing—who you are.

If we could self-reflect, we would understand our role in the world and how we could positively influence.

I want to provide a simple explanation that will give you the ability to formulate practical ways to accept or change who you are at your core self from a place of understanding and perspective.

Who you are is your identity—the way you look at yourself and relate to the world. Understanding this allows you to examine who you are and, more importantly, create who you want to be (if you feel unhappy with your perception of who you are).

It refers to the global understanding a person has of himself.

Self-identity is composed of permanent self-assessments, such as personality attributes, knowledge, skills and abilities, occupation, hobbies, and awareness of one's physical attributes.

The way you talk about yourself expresses your perception of yourself, but it is important to distinguish between self-concept and a temporary state.

For instance, the statement, "I am lazy" is a self-assessment that contributes to one's self-concept. In contrast, the statement "I am tired" would not usually be considered part of someone's self-concept since being tired is a temporary state.

The problem arises when we talk about ourselves with self-concept all the time. We do it irrationally, without noticing that we are recording this self-talk in our subconscious.

Self-identity is not restricted to the present. The future self or "possible self" represents your ideas of what you might become, what you would like to become, and what you are afraid of becoming. They correspond to hopes, fears, standards, goals, and threats.

The possible self may function as an incentive for future behavior and possibly evaluate oneself's current view.

Your boundaries are much the same as the boundary lines of a property. In a personal development sense, the boundaries are more difficult to see and be aware of. Still, in a nutshell, your boundaries include the preferences or rules you have about things, like what you will accept in behavior from and toward yourself, and your ability to say either yes or no to events or statements.

Another concept not excluded from self-identity is one's worldview, which refers to the structure or framework a person uses to organize and define what the world is to them. A person's worldview should allow them to understand how the world functions and how it is structured. It should encompass the totality, everything that exists around us, including the physical universe, the Earth, life and living things, mind, society, and culture.

We are an essential part of that world and the Universe, and our inner forces and energy are related. Therefore, a worldview should also answer the fundamental question: Who are we?

This question is essential because it will make you face a reality many people don't want to see.

People are used to defining themselves by their work, profession, beliefs, relationships, or other affiliations. Still, no matter what method of self-definition you choose, they are all subject to misinterpretation. Everyone has biases, and those biases will reflect the way a person interprets your self-description. For instance, if you describe yourself as a person who does not believe in someone superior's spiritual existence, others would interpret you automatically as an atheist because many people, especially religious people, do not know the true definition of "agnostic."

Calling yourself an atheist introduces a new set of problems. Instead of people mistakenly thinking that you are one of those "spiritual but not religious" people, they assume that you worship the devil when you do not believe in the devil, either!.

My point is that the way you define yourself will be interpreted differently by everyone. If you use categorizations to describe yourself, be prepared to elaborate on your self-description, and clarify confusing points.

All this chaos or entropy can be avoided (or it will be dissipated) if you null, thwart, or oppose the labeling and categorizing yourself.

You are not Mr. "The Doctor" or Ms. The Architect. You are YOU.

The name given to you at birth is what defines you as a child, teen, and adult. A title, condition, expertise, or background is not who you are—it is what you have achieved during your existence.

Maintain your sense of self; don't let anyone tell you who you are. *You* define who you are. We have already accepted several limitations as truths. Some of these limitations are real, but living in them is something we choose.

Belief systems or philosophies are also a misleading way to define yourself. Every belief system contains a set of values. When you describe yourself using a belief system, you express their values, not yours.

People subscribe to belief systems that support their existing values. In my humble opinion, this is why there are so many religions (and variants of these religions). Back in the day, someone disagreed with how someone else interpreted the Bible, or the Torah, or the Tripitaka / Pali Canon. Then other religions were created based on new interpretations.

When a person finds that a belief system no longer reflects their core value, they must decide. They must either modify their core value or find a new belief system.

If you are defined by a type of philosophy or belief system, at this moment, you will end up losing identity and live confused about who you are, in essence.

We spend so much time living our lives based on how others define us, either living by those standards or spending all our time setting up dogged philosophical fences against them. We develop heartfelt explanations and ideals around all those standards we do not want. So why is it that, instead of pursuing our own thing, we live framed by others?

There are two questions you have to be able to answer to yourself: "Who are you?" and "Why should someone care about you?"

It sounds very harsh, but no one cares about you—not, at least, at first. You need to *make* them care about you, and you will accomplish this with the way you define yourself.

Aristotle said, "It is the mark of an educated mind to be able to entertain a thought without accepting it."

You can agree or disagree with philosophies, beliefs, customs, traditions, living styles, thoughts, etc. However, you don't need to make them your mainstay where you sustain your existence, nor do you need to define yourself by them.

Some people get confused if they can't follow the norm and name who they are.

You need to create peace of mind and meaning that works for you.

Allocate a place accordingly where you want to be. Make a conscious decision to live life in a specific way that works for you best, not influenced by beliefs or philosophies imposed during your childhood programming or domestication.

You don't need people to understand who you are or what you do. You don't need other people's acceptance and validation. You only need to understand and accept yourself. Only then will people accept you for who you are.

Once you know who you are and accept who you are, people will perceive a structure and pattern and are more likely to accept it. Now that you know you don't need their acceptance for your existence, they will probably use you as a mirror to validate and identify themselves. It is from those points of coincidences that their acceptance will come from.

A definition of who you are creates a story, and stories are good.

The story tells who you are, what you do, why you are doing that, and what happened since you started living your journey. It makes you attractive, and it makes you valuable, and it teaches other people about you without influencing their perception and visual perspective of you.

Affirm who you are from your origin, from your childhood, and a perspective free of programming.

Attractive people are drawn to interesting people.

Stability and structure are fundamental to organize your life and disperse the entropy. It is best to build your routines and structure your life based on who you are. Build activities, habits, and values on something defined, instead of on clutter or chaos.

We are capable of amazing things, but "amazing" is about taking the second step. We free ourselves when we start challenging our limitations.

Freedom lies in choice—every time you choose to begin a new story for yourself, that is empowerment. Every time you choose without outside influence what you eat or how you dress, you are liberating yourself. When you begin to change, you stop destroying your life and start building it from absolute freedom.

Our worldview is our standard of how things are or should be in the world we live immersed. It is a global concept that makes up our values and morals, our rules of how we and others should act, relate, and operate within the world. Most people's worldviews are a vague set of rules and guidelines that have been unconsciously adopted from life experiences and influences. We adopted these rules from our friends, family, religious groups, and society but seldom took on the active process of creating our own.

We can create aspects of our worldview through our intellect, using rational and conscious decisions or emotionally charged ideas and concepts. Our worldviews are filters through which we make judgments of others and ourselves. The way we relate to the world and our behavior with it is the mirror reflection of how we relate to ourselves. It's time to fix our worldview, clean it, beautify it, to reflect the results in our own lives. Your ability to say yes or no to consumption habits has a primordial role in saving the planet and, therefore, your own life.

Our entire planet is suffocated, exhausted, depleted of resources, and collapsed, and we are doing hardly anything to fix the damage we have done. Moreover, we continue to contribute to its destruction without considering that what we are causing is our destruction and the extinction of The Planet.

We have come a long way in the last centuries of humanity. Some things are obsolete and need to be adapted, changed, or modified to adjust to today's reality.

Self-awareness has become a powerful weapon against human misery.

There is no higher vibrational state than being in tune with your true self. Knowing who you are and what you genuinely want is a potent tool for personal growth and life transformation. Keep this knowledge at the forefront of your brain by spending a little time each day focusing on it.

Having a clear and defined rule for yourself about the worldview you and others should live will make you distinguish luxury from necessity and an appropriate relationship from a deceptive relationship with the world.

You need to define limit preferences and say "no" to some requests about this worldview rule. The media, society, and the people around you will try to manipulate you or press your buttons. They will say things that will try to hurt you, drive you, confuse you—but you will not be affected.

If you have a concrete rule about this, when they push you, they will feel the resistance: your steadfastness, your resolve, and your boundaries.

And while these people may not like your decision, they will respect you for it and will know they cannot get what they want out of you.

You will have encountered a situation that will remain true to who you are. You will feel good about yourself. Because you followed your worldview rules, you will fill yourself with self-esteem a little more, and it will strengthen your self-identity.

To conclude, the essential points to remember are:

- Define who you are, but don't let anyone attempt to provide an answer on your behalf.
- Find a clear and defined rule for yourself about your worldview.
- Set up a lifestyle accordingly.
- Develop self-awareness because it is a powerful weapon against human misery.

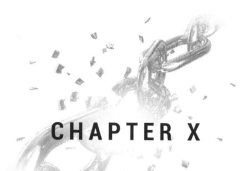

CHAPTER X

Reborn and Flourishing

Being reborn is about developing understanding, awareness, enlightenment, insight, and wisdom. It is learning about the unknown and applying knowledge of the lessons learned but staying open-minded. It is about advancement, development, open-mindedness, culture, refinement, and cultivation. It will lead you to a new life.

Let me introduce you to a new version of yourself built up with strong self-esteem.

Self-esteem is perhaps the single most crucial emotional gauge of our ability to feel almost all other positive emotions and beliefs about ourselves. It affects our measure of happiness, success, well-being, confidence, and assurance.

While self-esteem is a general state of mind, it is affected by changes in any of the various feelings that make it up. We learned already how mood changes could relate directly to the way you eat, exercise, and sleep, influencing neurotransmitters' production, functionality, and mental clarity. Al these factors are the pure reflection of our lifestyle.

A drop in confidence will lower self-esteem in the short term. A prolonged negative experience will produce a longer-term reduction of self-esteem.

Positive emotional experiences will increase the sensation. In simple terms, when you experience an event or situation that supports your worldview, your esteem increases—and vice versa.

Understanding where you are now will give you the clarity needed to develop a new plan for your life. It does not have to be perfectly planned because you won't have all the answers you are looking for. It will not be as if you have opened a book and read the solutions for your problems, but rather like a process of awareness, where you will encounter enlightenment to wisdom.

Take the time to sit down in a quiet place. Focus your attention to develop a map of your life to the detail. Visualize the life you want to have, the person you want to become, the path you want to walk, the places you want to visit, the way you want to live.

Apply the wisdom you have acquired over the years to realize the way you are driving your life. Realize who you are today compared with who you were yesterday, starting from your origin.

Get your gloves on and get to work! Reading this book (or any other book) and not applying anything you have learned won't change anything in your life. Work on the areas of your life that are not working for you. Your relationship with yourself comes first, then other areas of your life where you sense discomfort and can't interact the way you would like. Most of the time, these discomfort areas fix instantly after your relationship with yourself is in harmony.

The way you physically look and how you expose yourself to your world can be distorted from your perspective and the world's perception of you. It is not a bad thing—on the contrary. The world can appreciate many of your beauties that you are blinded to.

Discover your inner beauty. We are all beautiful inside. We all have a light to shine.

Fall in love with your inner beauty and get used to seeing it in the mirror. The inner beauty is the real beauty of a person that goes far beyond just physical appearances.

It is what someone experiences through another person's character and personality. You may assume that inner beauty is something you can only feel and never see, but how true is that? You may think that you never notice inner beauty at first sight. Almost all the time, we notice a person's physical appearance only for a moment, until the real inner beauty starts the attraction game.

You may speak to someone for a minute and find them pleasant or not-so-pleasant at first, but you may start to pick up on their qualities and traits as the conversation goes on. Without even realizing it, you may begin to find a person more and more beautiful or charming. Outer beauty only works for a glance. It's inner beauty that makes someone stay. We have overlooked the real inner beauty and given all the credit to outer beauty.

Why do some people glow more than others?

More than anything else, it is a person's inner belief that they are attractive, making them more appealing to others.

It's true, and I cannot deny it—physical appearances can be a bonus, but it is something that's easily overlooked when other traits are brought into the picture.

The glow of confidence and self-belief comes from within and makes you attractive to everybody.

First impressions don't always depend on your physique or facial features, but you need to believe that from within yourself. That's where your true beauty lies.

Are you beautiful on the inside? Of course, you are! More than you appreciate.

If you love, appreciate, and feel good about yourself, you will feel more confident when interacting with other people, and you will attract other beautiful people into your life. When we fill our thoughts with positive energy and inner beauty, we appreciate the things surrounding us.

Even if we look at an inanimate object like a painting or a view of the ocean, it will look more beautiful because we see the beauty overflows within us, reflecting on everything else around us.

Everyone only sees you as a projection of what you see when you look into the mirror. You're beautiful if you know it and feel it. So go on out there, because there's a whole world waiting for the beautiful you. And if you still feel like there's a flaw holding the beautiful you back, learn to overcome it.

No one is perfect, and no one ever will be. We all have flaws to burnish and sides to improve. Even the person most similar to perfection has several areas in which to improve. Nobody is perfect. It is what I call the beauty of imperfection!

So far, we have developed several topics that may have served as informative help or general knowledge, but nothing you have read will make your life transform to what you want if you do not get down to work.

The next chapter is the first step to take, of many other steps you will have to take down, to start a new path that will lead you to a change in your life.

As I mentioned at the beginning of this book, several careers and professions came into my life for a reason. One of them was Vegan Chef, so as a chef, I will give you my Detox Plan.

This detoxification plan has been followed by many people who reversed many different health problems, but you don't have to have a condition to follow this diet; you just need the will to improve your health and the way you live today.

The way we feed ourselves is key to proper functioning.

The last chapter is full of step-by-step recipes designed to clean your body, help your body repair cell damage, and live an abundant, harmonious life.

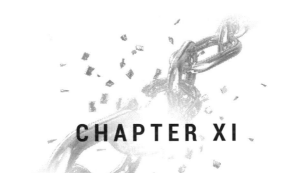

CHAPTER XI

A Change in Lifestyle - Recipes for the soul

Life blooms with the flow of giving and receiving. Nothing is static. Our bodies flourish with the dynamic of constant exchange with the universe's forces: energy and entropy.

There must exist cooperation between each other. Nature provides us with a perfect symphony: the sun provides warmth for seeds to sprout, rain brings the needed moisture for crops, and these crops subsequently will give the food that will nourish our bodies.

Nowhere in the natural world does "holding" exist. The process of giving and receiving is a crucial part of nature's rich abundance. The easiest way to get what you want is by giving others what they need. The more you give, the more you receive.

All life events are governed by the law of cause and effect, giving us freedom of choice. If we don't like the results of the previous selection, we can always choose again.

In every situation, countless alternatives can affect you, and some can wound you. When you make one particular choice, it will have consequences that will affect you and those surrounding you for good or bad.

It will sound repetitive but, responsibly care for something you value as part of realizing your dreams. Take proper care of yourself and your loved ones, make healthy choices for your body, and use all-natural resources responsibly.

"Freedom lies in choices responsible taken." *-Ana Fessia-*

Let me transport you to an unknown place. Close your eyes and stimulate your senses with aromas that bring you happy memories. How could you not enjoy the scent of fresh mint leaves in a homemade lemonade? How could you not delight with the refreshing aroma of orange zest?!

This chapter is about falling in love with real, healthy food. It is designed to introduce you to *"Recipes for the Soul,"* my next upcoming book. Connect with your senses. Awaken and engage with the world. Open your eyes to discover the true colors of nature.

We spoke in past chapters about the importance of food. What we eat interferes with our daily performance, our feelings, and our mood.

In the beginning, I mentioned that some people develop chronic diseases such as diabetes, high blood pressure, cholesterol, depression, psoriasis, thyroidism, cancer, autoimmune diseases like lupus, and obesity because of the lifestyle and diets.

What we eat is our fuel. If we choose the wrong food, the machine (our body) becomes the catalyst for problems—and provides the perfect environment (like acidosis) for diseases to arise.

What I'm about to share with you has helped many people reverse many of those diseases. Every person's immune system is different, and results vary based (mainly) on the person's will, commitment, and perseverance—just like everything else in life.

Let's start from the most precious moment of everyday life: the moment when we open our eyes and wake up from a peaceful night to get ready to begin a new day.

We never think about the preciousness of that present second when our body wakes up.

Our body is ready to start a new day! Our brain is connecting back with reality. During sleep time, most of our organs had repaired cellular damage, and millions of metabolic processes, biological functions, and chemical reactions had occurred during sleep time.

All the hard work the body did during the time we were resting released residuals or ashes that resulted from chemical combustions. Those ashes increased the amount of acidity in our bodies.

Every time we sleep, our body will work hard to fix problems here and there. The immune system has an essential role in this task because it will defend our cells from pathogens and other harmful substances.

Suppose our diet is not anti-inflammatory, and most of the food we consume is processed food high in saturated fats, sugars, sodium, and bad carbs. In that case, we are developing a perfect environment for any chronic disease. Simultaneously, we are creating a lot of acidity and inflammation; And widespread inflammation is a very unfavorable situation.

What we eat is vital. If we eat processed foods, the immune system will be busy and focused on defending the body from what we have eaten. Instead of receiving the nutrients to repair cell damage and decrease inflammation, the immune system will be fighting against the chemical compounds in processed food.

Let's focus on how to help our body in its never-ending work.

The first thing we must do in the morning before getting out of bed is to stretch our body and oxygenate our brain, breathing deeply in and exhaling deeply out. Do this at least three times.

Smile, be grateful and feel the joy of having another day to live in front of you.

Next, go to the kitchen and prepare a big glass of warm water with lemon juice (one whole lemon) and drink it right away. It will help your body eliminate the acidity produced during the night.

After that, you can start your daily routine. Shower, get dressed, and so on.

I like to go for a short walk with my dog to activate my muscles and then spend twenty to thirty minutes at the gym or exercising at home. You can find thousands of good videos online, where people post their training sessions. It's a fun and varied way to exercise.

I prefer outdoor activities because, at the same time, I'm exercising, I'm also helping my body synthesize vitamin D and absorb vitamin C.

There will always be excuses to avoid exercise, but once you get used to set the clock forty-five minutes before the time you are used to waking up, you will discover they are the most priceless forty-five minutes in the day. If you are not a morning person, you can set those forty-five minutes in the afternoon, before dinner time.

Back home, you can start a detox plan to complement your daily exercise routine. This detox plan has helped many people, and now, I will give it to you as a gift!

TWENTY-ONE DAYS DETOX PLAN

First, we are going to prepare four green smoothies. They will provide us with all the energy needed to start our day in optimum conditions.

We will drink these smoothies gradually during the morning, starting with the first one right after exercising.

Breakfast: Green smoothies can be with or without bananas. Bananas are an excellent source of potassium and fructose. It will help you start the day full of energy. You can alternate and prepare two with and two without bananas if you like.

If you want your smoothies with bananas, in a powerful blender, put four ripe bananas, two full hands of spinach, one full hand of kale, one frozen, ripe banana, one full hand of frozen berries, and two glasses of cold water. Blend until getting a creamy and smooth preparation.

If you want your smoothies without bananas, in a blender, put one cucumber, two celery stalks, two full hands of spinach, one full hand of kale, one whole peeled lemon, one full hand of parsley, and one peeled and seeded green apple or a cup of ripe pineapple chunks. Divide the smoothie into four mason jars and save it in a refrigerator or carry it with you to work in a refrigerated lunchbox.

Pack your lunch; For lunch, you can have a big salad made of all kinds of raw veggies and greens, with a homemade dressing: blend cilantro, avocado, and lemon juice with a pinch of Pink Himalayan salt and a bit of water to make it liquid enough but still creamy.

Add to the lunchbox one snack: fresh fruit of your choice, cut into cubes. The amount is not limited. You can eat four apples or a whole watermelon. Eat until you are satisfied with that only fruit, what I called a "mono-meal."

When you come back from work, prepare a fruit smoothie with two fruits of your preference. It can be two ripe bananas and (fresh or frozen) strawberries; bananas and blueberries; two oranges and strawberries, watermelon and mint leaves, or honeydew and mint leaves.

For dinner, you will bake chopped veggies. Combine any of your preferences, like sweet potato, butternut squash, red peppers, onion, garlic, broccoli, cauliflower, zucchini, spinach, mushroom, Brussel sprouts, asparagus, and so on. You can choose any veggies except regular potatoes, eggplant, and green peppers because they contain nightshades and aren't good during the detox process.

Drink plenty of water and herbal teas without caffeine during the day.

Have at least two freshly squeezed juices(or smoothies) with five of any of the following ingredients: beet, carrot, green apples, celery, cucumber, orange, pineapple, kiwi, and papaya. Do not combine more than five ingredients at one time. The best combination is four vegetables (at least three greens) and one fruit, but you can always add a full peeled lemon and a piece of ginger to any of the combinations.

My preferred juice is cucumber, parsley, celery, spinach, and green apple. I add a full peeled lemon and a tip of a thumb of fresh ginger root. You can alternate, and instead of spinach, use kale, sometimes. You can drink juices as afternoon snacks or, if you prefer, you can have one type of freshly cut fruit (another mono-meal)

I recommend you to be committed to yourself and steady with this diet through no less than twenty-one days. Everything we do uninterruptedly for twenty-one days or more becomes a habit.

During the first week you can eat soups and cooked veggies for dinner, but don't eat anything other than vegetables and fruits. If it is not a fruit or a veggie, do not touch it! No processed vegan food or processed vegetables, or frozen vegan dinners. Only fresh, natural ingredients.

During the second week, cut to half the cooked dinners and eat more raw. Let's say three days of cooked food for dinner and four days of raw food for dinner. You will find a ton of recipes online if you search for raw vegan dishes. Do not be tempted by the delicious desserts you will find. You must stay away from foods like walnuts, cashews, coconut oil, coconut milk, and almond milk during those twenty-one days because we are looking for a fat-free detox. Even though these nuts are great for your health, they create interaction with the immune system during the detox process. We don't want that. We are trying to give the immune system a break and focus on repair damage and reducing inflammation.

For the third week, try to go fully raw. The change will be stunning! If it is too hard, you can add some cooked warm food at night, like a veggie soup.

If you need extra energy during the day, you can add one or two dates to your smoothies and no more than half an avocado a day to your salads. Avoid oils in your salad dressings. You can use one teaspoon of olive oil a day.

Check out these three options for salad dressings:

First option: Blend lemon juice, half an avocado, cilantro, Himalayan salt, and water.

Second option: Blend sun-dried tomato, basil leaves, one garlic clove, rice vinegar, one tablespoon of olive oil, Himalayan salt, and water.

Third option: Blend one bunch of fresh basil leaves, one garlic clove, one tablespoon of olive oil, rice vinegar, one teaspoon of agave, Himalayan salt, and water.

With these three variations, you won't miss any other salad dressing.

As you can see by going through the reading, living a simple life is easy. What makes it complicated is us! Go back to your roots.

Become the seed nurtured by the fertile soil, and then flourish with love.

Go back and read those chapters that connect with your situation and inner voice as many times as you need.

Make a list of those things you would like to improve or change. Keep records of the evolution of your desires and take accountability for your steps toward those desires. Track your life's journey. Write a diary, starting with gratitude for another day full of opportunities.

Smile when you wake up, laugh frequently, and think positive when storms arrive in your life. Change your perspective and consider difficulties as lessons and growth opportunities.

Be generous, kind, and compassionate. Let others love you, but most importantly, love yourself. With every change in values comes identity crises, chaos, or entropy, hence re-definement and direction change. This is all part of growth.

We have reached the end of this journey together. We have shared many moments, maybe hours, connected by the book. In every word you read, my soul and I were there with you. When you finish this book, we no longer will be together, sharing that space and those moments. We will separate for a moment, but my love and gratitude to you will still be there. While we may not have met face to face, we have touched hearts, feelings, emotions, and thoughts.

We leave each other full of practical and simple tools we can apply in our lives to improve those aspects with which we disagree.

I have sincere and deep gratitude to you for allowing me to share part of my life and experience. My sincere hope is that something I have shared here has taken you to that special place you were looking for.

Stay connected with me—write me a few lines telling me about your experience and the path traveled to achieve full happiness. I look forward to meeting you and hearing about your life's success story. Life crosses paths in many ways. At least for now, we have traveled this path together!

"Life is a fleeting moment that fits in a sigh, in the blink of an eye, in a look, in a smile.

Do not let that priceless moment pass unnoticed in the eyes of those who love you and share the journey with you.

Trace a footprint, leave a message, and plant a seed for the earth that housed you with love."

Ana Fessia

May life fill you with blessings!

Thank you!

Contact the Author:

Instagram: https://www.instagram.com/ana.fessia2020/

Facebook: https://www.facebook.com/ana.fessia

Email: ana.fessia07@gmail.com